CHEATS AND EATS
LIFESTYLE PROGRAMME

CHEATS AND EATS
LIFESTYLE PROGRAMME

Eat the Foods You Crave and Lose Weight Even Faster

Jackie Wicks with Rob Hobson

Cheats and Eats Lifestyle Programme

Published and cover design by:
 Healthspan
Healthspan House
The Grange
St Peter Port
Guernsey
GY1 2QH

Author Biographies

Jackie Wicks, founder of PEERtrainer, creator and author of the Cheats & Eats Lifestyle Programme

JACKIE WICKS, founder of PEERtrainer, is the creator of the Cheats and Eats Lifestyle programme, an entirely new diet system using carefully vetted experts, technology expertise and the PEERtrainer community to nail the support piece of dieting and help people successfully follow through. PEERtrainer is an innovative online support system with 75,000,000 unique visitors since launch with members losing 50, 60 and even 100 pounds. US News & World Report calls PEERtrainer one of the best sites to lose weight, and it's been featured on *Good Morning America*, *PEOPLE* magazine, *The New York Times*, *The Wall Street Journal*, *USA Today*, *O* magazine and *Good Housekeeping*.

Rob Hobson, Registered Nutritionist (BSc Nutrition) (MSc Public Health Nutrition) (AFN) – Healthspan's Head of Nutrition and UK consultant on the Cheats and Eats Lifestyle Programme

Rob is one of the UK's most well-respected and highly trained nutritionists. He has worked in public health for government agencies, charity organisations and the NHS. Rob is a prominent figure within the media working on TV and radio, and writing extensively across the media for many top health and fitness publications, websites and news outlets. Rob continues to work as a consultant for health and fitness companies worldwide as well as working privately with celebrities and other high-profile clients.

Nicola Addison, Health, Fitness & Well-being Expert. Creator of the Cheats & Eats workout

With over 18 years of successful industry experience in some of the UK's most prestigious wellness centres, Nicola currently provides consultancy services to brands, businesses and individuals in the UK and Europe.

Nicola is a well-known industry voice and regularly publishes across the national press. Her work includes brand representation, public speaking, written content and press tips.

A Foreword By
Tim Pethick, Healthspan CEO

Healthspan is a company that creates supplements. But we have a core belief that underpins our approach to everything we do. Better living needn't be elusive; health and happiness are what life's all about. We believe the quality of your life as you age is, to a great extent, under your control. Achieving this long, healthy lifespan (healthspan) comes from focusing on three key pillars – staying active, eating well and being positive. We exist to supplement and support you in achieving these things.

Earlier this year we launched our 'NutriCoach' personalised nutrition ecosystem of activity tracker, smart body composition scales, and app with food logging, daily health scoring and smart recommendations for micronutrient supplementation, hydration and protein support. One of the things we learned from early customers of this coaching system is that almost all of them begin their journey to better health by wanting to lose some weight.

Most of us tackle weight loss using diet and exercise and, for me, both are crucial in finding the perfect balance in life. They work hand-in-hand to ensure overall health and well-being. However, our relationship with food and exercise is often a rocky one that is far from being straight forward.

We are surrounded by diets and food fads, all claiming to be the holy grail of weight loss. But for every story about a new diet craze there is a story debunking an old one or profiling those who just couldn't sustain their diet.

Diet can be seen as a comprise to your lifestyle but actually, it doesn't have to be. I was determined to find a solution that was built on the foundations of our three pillars – stay active, eat well and be positive. It should be possible to help people achieve the perfect equilibrium between diet and exercise, without having to compromise on a normal lifestyle.

During my search, I came across Jackie Wicks, founder of PEERtrainer, a lifestyle programme that is far from being your regular diet. Jackie's approach, based on an understanding that we can't be perfect all the time, was to create a system of diet, exercise and positivity that is sustainable and therefore enduring. Jackie's cheat system has proven to be very successful in the US, where Jackie is from. It was the voice of reason I was looking for that really resonated with Healthspan's key beliefs of living a healthy and long lifespan.

Jackie's emphasis on eating healthily and staying active permanently, rather than just in the short term, is evident throughout this book which is why, with our support, this is just the beginning of your quest to be the best version of yourself that you can possibly be.

You'll have heard the common phrase 'you are what you eat' and, this is true. We want to help people who've come to that realisation and to make a change. No one is perfect and if you want to improve then a sympathetic guide to help is essential.

Healthspan (www.healthspan.co.uk) are the UK's leading online direct supplier of vitamins, supplements and are here to support you with all your health and well-being goals. The Cheats and Eats system is soon to be incorporated into the Healthspan NutriCoach app, check the website for release date details.

Contents

Introduction: Why You Can't Lose Weight Now   *1*

Part One: Easy Is Better Than Hard   9

1. Why Cheating Will Help You Finally Succeed   11
   Why You're Doing Everything "Right" but Nothing
   Is Working

2. Why You Lose When You Cheat and Eat   26
   Stop Counting Calories/Fat/Fibre/Sugar/Nutrients,
   Stop Eating Too Little, Stop Obsessing – and Stop
   Going Up and Down on the Scale

3. Move More – The Non Negotiable!   53
   How You Work Out, Stress Out, and Lose Nothing –
   and Why Cheating Will "Work Out" for You

Part Two: Lose Weight, Fast   81

4. The Cheats and Eats Lifestyle Programme
   Explained   82
   Eats: You Can Never Be Too Rich, Too Thin, or Eat
   Too Many Eats
   Cheats: Keep All the Foods You Love to Eat, Just
   Limit the Cheats

5. The Cheats and Eats Lifestyle Programme
Week One   110
Eat the Eats, and You Have 10 Cheats

6. The Cheats and Eats Lifestyle Programme
Week Two   119
Eat the Eats and Earn More Cheats

7. The Cheats and Eats Lifestyle Programme
Week Three   127
Eat the Eats, Learn to Cheat

8. Your Magic Fridge   134
How to Buy and Cook Smart

Part Three: Cheaters for Life   143

9. The Cheating Gourmet   144
*How to Create a Magic Kitchen (With over 100
Recipes for Cheating and Eating!)*

10. The Cheats and Eats Lifestyle Programme
Maintenance Plan   278
How to Keep the Weight You've Lost Off – For Good

Conclusion: Why You Can Lose Weight Now   286

Appendix   290

Useful Measurements   293

Bibliography   298

Index   302

Introduction: Why You Can't Lose Weight Now

Welcome. We are so excited to share The Cheats and Eats Lifestyle Programme with you because we know you'll find relief in these pages. There is a lot of pain and frustration out there for people who are struggling with their weight; We hear it every day. Dieting has become so confusing, regimented and contradictory. People often put all their faith into the promises made by the latest trendy diet but are frequently left with an overwhelming feeling of failure when t hey become defeated within days of trying something new or even before they start. I personally receive daily emails and hear from readers that say, "I've already cheated this morning. My day is shot. What's the point?"

I used to think the same thing. I would get up, be late, need "energy" for a meeting and get a bacon-egg-and-cheese sandwich and a large latte. In that moment, I would think, "Ugh, I cheated again." And I would beat myself up. I wanted to lose weight so badly. I was determined to get back into my pre-pregnancy clothes – so why was I unable to stick to eating healthily?

It took me a long time to realise and understand that the most important thing to remember about weight loss is that there should always be some room for mistakes and slip-ups. Beating myself up over a mistake at breakfast didn't get me anywhere and thinking that I had failed often meant giving up completely leading to more bad choices at lunch, or giving me an excuse to skip the gym and hang out on the sofa.

So, I started to think, What could work? What could I actually do? What plan would actually work? What diet plan could I do where I could lose weight and still go out to dinner and eat without feeling guilty? What would people like me actually do, not just for one week, not just for two weeks, not just for three weeks? What would people like me actually do, day in and day out, without getting frustrated or discouraged the moment they slipped up by having cheese and crackers?

When people cheat on their diets, they quit. But they still desperately want a plan that works – one that helps them lose weight and get healthy. Any plan that works in real life must keep people from quitting. A plan that works in real life must allow for slip-ups, cheats, making mistakes and room to enjoy birthday parties or social occasions with your friends.

I've spent many years obsessed with one question: What diet will people actually follow through with? People want to stick to a programme and achieve their weight and health goals, and I wanted to find the diet that will help them actually do it. I've been obsessed with finding the combination of habits and practices that will help people commit to losing weight, being healthy, feeling good and getting rid of the guilt.

If most popular diet and fitness regimens actually worked, we wouldn't be continually frustrated and have such an impossible time losing weight. The information many of these diet regimes provide isn't bad. The problem is that most of these programmes are easy when you're psyched or motivated. But what about when you're not? Any barrier to change no matter how small is likely to impact on your motivation to lose weight. When you're overwhelmed or stressed? When your boss hands you something at 5 p.m.? When you get in a fight with a sibling? When your babysitter cancels? Or maybe you just have one of those days when nothing seems to be going the way you want. Then the rules seem impossible and you end up saying those fateful words to yourself, "I'll start tomorrow". That's when we resort to our old habits that won't help us lose weight, but ultimately, are easy – and we need easy when the tsunami of the world overwhelms us.

Whatever the plan is – even if it has the best information available – if you don't put it into action it might as well just be a movie. Afterwards you think, "Wow, that looked really great. Wish I could do that/go there/be that person." That's why I'm obsessed with follow-through. The most successful diet is always going to be the one that you can stick to and we know you will be able to stick to The Cheats and Eats Lifestyle Programme, thousands of people have already.

What you'll learn in this book may be the opposite of what some people think "works" for weight loss. For example, you'll learn that **portion control can't work alone** – because most of the time, people can't follow through no matter how well intentioned.

If people feel hungry, they'll "cheat" and feel so guilty, they quit. The truth, as you'll learn in the next chapter, is that you only have to monitor how much you eat of some foods, not everything you eat. **You can eat as much as you want of many foods and still lose weight!**

So, what's my story and why should you take advice from me? In 2004, I was a new mum of a baby boy, and I realised I had only lost twenty pounds from the peak of my pregnancy weight, which was just over 13 stone. (I'm five foot five.) After months of being at 11st 7lb, it was evident that I wasn't going to be one of the lucky ones for whom breastfeeding took off the weight. I was so frustrated I knew what I had to do, but I just wasn't doing it. My good friend Jen and I started emailing our daily food and workout habits back and forth to provide the accountability we needed. Two other friends joined us and the first "PEERtrainer group" was born.

One year later, I founded a website called PEERtrainer.com to help people who knew how to lose weight but had a tough time following through (like me). Since then, PEERtrainer has become the premier online weight-loss lab in the US, with over 75,000,000 unique visitors since our launch over a decade ago. Experts from every discipline approach us, write for us and partner with us in order to deliver their most cutting-edge health information to our community. We bring this to the world every day. I see the problems and struggles people have with dieting because I personally read every email that comes in – and most of the struggles and problems are ones I have experienced too. I know how people succeed and what contributes to their failures. Through mine and other peoples shared experiences, I have learnt exactly what works and what doesn't.

The foundation of The Cheats and Eats Lifestyle Programme is the Cheats and Eats sheet. When the Cheats and Eats Lifestyle Programme

> The only diet and exercise regimen that works is the one you'll actually do – a plan you'll follow through on.

was first created, it was just a simple list with very little explanation, a few recipes, and some gentle motivation. We didn't create a three-week plan. We didn't create a meal plan or an exercise plan.

We gave our members the basics because we wanted to see how the PEERtrainer community would respond – but also, more importantly, how our members would work with the list. Would they find it doable? Would they lose weight? What parts would they find confusing and what parts would they love?

Over 100,000 people downloaded our simple, 26-page PDF. After about a year, we surveyed our community to find out how they did with it. By just doing the basics, members had an average one stone weight loss over a three-month period. We learned not only was the The Cheats and Eats Lifestyle Programme doable, it was also successful – and everyone was asking for a full plan. This book is that full plan.

The Cheats and Eats Lifestyle Programme is simple. It's a list of "Eats" (foods that will help you lose weight) and "Cheats" (foods that hinder weight loss). We take out complicated calculations, we convince you that starving yourself won't work, and we make it so food doesn't drive you crazy. You're no longer consumed by the thought of how you're going to get through a lunch with co-workers or that "obligation" meals at your in-laws. The Cheats and Eats Lifestyle Programme builds on what you already know – that some foods are great for you, and others aren't – by giving you a super-easy way to think about eating, incorporating exercise and enjoying life into your diet. We make it easy for you to lose weight without restricting any food from your diet.

Some diet and exercise experts focus on the science of losing weight: nutrition, cortisol, hormones, etc. Others zero in on exercise. Some diets concentrate on every calorie you eat. Some focus on nutrients. Some emphasise on eliminating entire food groups. And though all of these factors may have a hand in weight loss, what's most important is *finding the plan that you'll do* – and that won't cause the same frustration most of us feel with certain diets.

Most people I talk to don't want the über buff-body or have huge muscles (and if you are one of those people, inspired by growth hormone and testosterone-filled bodies, this book is not for you). Most of us don't want to sacrifice our time with our family or friends to hours in the gym. We just want to look good and feel good. We just want to go shopping and find an outfit that looks great – and not have to have to try on fifty different things, just to find something that fits. We want energy. We want health. We want to not be tired all the time.

Many diet and exercise plans are extremely regimented and sure, if you follow them to the letter, you'll have that perfect body they promise. But because we don't necessarily want to sacrifice living our lives to become that perfect specimen of health and fitness, we can't follow those plans exactly, and this can leave us feeling guilty or that we have failed in some way. The Cheats and Eats Lifestyle Programme lets you keep the foods you love, stops the guilt about your third glass of wine and gives you a simple way to live your life.

We get that you might feel guilty about the wedge of cheese that you ate, the missed workouts and your chocolate habit. We get that if you're a parent – especially if you're a mum – you sometimes feel like you're a slave to your family without any time to yourself.

We've all woken up on a Monday morning, thinking, "This is it, today is the day I'm going to start." And then your husband asks, "Hey babe, where are my keys?" and the kids are running late for school, next thing you know all those barriers start to get in the way again; you're roped into a 10-minute search, everybody is running late, and there is no time for anything you wanted to do, whether it was an early-morning workout, making a healthy breakfast or packing your lunch.

Most of the people who preach about "making health a priority" or harangue you to just "stick to your diet," or inform you that what you really need is to pay a personal trainer to get in shape, often have no idea what it's like to live in the real world. But I do and I know what it's like to want to lose weight, to feel like you're doing *everything* right but nothing is working.

Maybe you are the 38-year-old mum who was skinny in her twenties but can't get back to that weight, or the 60-year-old woman who has the time to make healthy foods and eat a ton of vegetables but still doesn't see any success on the scale, or a 45-year-old father who is a vice president at his company and makes time to take care of his family, someone who understands exactly how to lose weight but just can't find time to do the workout. Or maybe you're the guy who woke up at 35 with a beer belly, suddenly two stone overweight and with no idea how you got there. Or maybe you're the person who is doing everything "right" according to what you see on TV and read in the health magazines but no matter what you do, the scale doesn't move. The Cheats and Eats Lifestyle Programme is for all of you.

We have spoken with leading health, nutrition and fitness experts, who have generously shared their expertise and knowledge with us for this book. I have also teamed up with one of the UK's leading nutritionists, Rob Hobson to write this edition of the book. Rob's enthusiasm, encyclopedic knowledge and experience of all things food and nutrition have provided valuable inspiration, insight and helped to put the science behind our plan.

The true power of The Cheats and Eats Lifestyle Programme comes from the feedback we get from the people following our plan. This valuable insight has shown us exactly what works and what doesn't. In this book, you'll finally learn why you're doing "everything right" and still can't lose the weight. Many people have shared stories with me that they wouldn't feel comfortable sharing with their husband or partner, friends, family members even their doctor. We have learnt their fears, their struggles, and their obstacles to losing weight. This is why The Cheats and Eats Lifestyle Programme works. And it works for life.

Here's How Monika from Atlanta Used The Cheats and Eats Lifestyle Programme

I used this system as my wedding diet. I went from 10st to 9st 4lb and felt wonderful for my wedding day. I think this works because it allows you to eat food from most food groups and not feel hungry. I would highly recommend it. You honestly feel better about doing this diet.

– Monika V

Your Secret Weapon

Even though you are living with loads of frustration, confusion and hopelessness that any diet solution will truly work, you have a secret weapon. Your secret weapon is an open mind. People who succeed on The Cheats and Eats Lifestyle Programme are open to ideas that may challenge the status quo, ideas that may be different than anything you have read or heard about before.

The Cheats and Eats Lifestyle Programme gives people a clear direction and it also gives people permission to *go at their own pace*. Often we are told that we have a "responsibility" to make dramatic changes, or that we just need to "make your health a priority." While these sentiments are well intended and do sometimes trigger the change you're trying for, often our brains will resist this – usually in a big way

According to Dr. Srini Pillay of the Harvard Medical School, our brains are built for slow and steady change, "Habit is the king that rules the brain. New habits must be nurtured in a steady manner." We want you to move toward the way of eating that works, *at your own pace*. We've learned that people *love* having freedom, especially when it comes to what they put on their plates.

That freedom paired with the plan that you can incorporate into your life helps rewire your brain over time – making change easier for you to follow through on.

Stop following all the diets you say you're going to do, knowing that you can't possibly do them in real life. Don't start the diet that makes you give up bread if you know that the second you do give up on bread, you'll want to eat an entire loaf. Stop counting every single crumb that goes in your mouth and stop stressing out when you can't possibly know how much fibre is in your food at dinner. Stop making it hard for yourself.

The Cheats and Eats Lifestyle Programme is forgiving but most important, flexible. *Nothing* is off the table. Join the hundreds of thousands of people who have had success with understanding how to lose weight without beating yourself up, and who know that The Cheats and Eats Lifestyle Programme works. You can do this. You can lose the weight with The Cheats and Eats Lifestyle Programme. And you will!

PART ONE

Easy Is Better Than Hard

CHAPTER 1

Why Cheating Will Help You Finally Succeed

Accept what is. Let go of what was. Have faith in what will be.

If you're like most people, you've read all the books, you know what you should be eating and doing, and you have a great deal of knowledge about diet and fitness but you have a tough time following through. The diet and fitness world "helps" by giving us contradictory solutions, ridiculous gimmicks, and impossible standards – all of which are completely frustrating, counterproductive and unsuccessful. The popularity of social media has led to many people taking advice from enviably fit, healthy bloggers and other such 'gurus' with no official training in nutrition or first-hand experience of losing weight. What I hear time and time again from people trying to lose weight is that they've tried a bunch of different diets but nothing works – or nothing works for long. Succeeding at weight loss involves a lot of factors, both physiological and psychological. If a diet doesn't take into consideration both – and many do not – that diet has set you up to fail. Period.

The Cheats and Eats Lifestyle Programme helps you tackle all that has stopped you from losing weight in the past, and will help you at every level – food and exercise, your body and your brain – so you *will* succeed. I've done it for myself.

Welcome to what works.

You Haven't Failed Diets, Diets have Failed *You*

There are a million fads out there: go clean, do Paleo, go vegan, go gluten-free, go whole foods, do whatever your best friend's sister is doing or what you see Jennifer Aniston talking about in a magazine – but then you don't have time to shop and cook and produce the latest braised fennel or make your own home-made kefir or nut milk.

> I wake up and go, it would be so cool to be a vegan...gonna start today. And then, I fry bacon.
>
> – Tyra Banks

Or you hear about a certain kind of yoga or exercise class, and you think, "Maybe that's it!" But rustling up the motivation to get to that class can stress you out to the point that it doesn't even seem worth it to you anymore.

Exercise programmes that gain massive popularity in a flash like HIIT or CrossFit are basically the same as trendy diets such as Paleo: supposed magic-bullet solutions that in reality don't work for most of us. Like dieting, there is no such thing as a "one-size-fits-all" approach, we are all different. Could you succeed in the short term? Sure, but these programmes are tough and restrictive, which most people can't maintain over the long term.

This is why so many people quit these fad diets and exercise programmes over and over again. I did, too. I quit when it gets too rough on the treadmill. I quit sometimes when I'm just sick of eating healthy food and really want a slice of pizza. I know I'm not alone here!

There is a biological reason we quit, why we give up when something we're trying to do becomes too hard. It's called *homeostasis*, and it applies to both your body and your mind. Your body wants to be in balance, and when it knows it's not – say, because you're killing yourself doing two CrossFit workouts a day, or spending the day at your desk starving on a calorie-restriction diet – it will do whatever it can to get back into homeostasis, the place it feels balanced.

Because of that, I would argue that quitting is not always a bad thing. It means you have taken on too much, and your whole mind and body is shouting, "This is not going to work." And your body and mind are right. One of the best things you can do is listen to your body because it will let you know when something is just not working for you.

Designed for people who have quit before, The Cheats and Eats Lifestyle Programme promotes balance. It makes your body happy and it's doable. The trick is to keep your body in homeostasis. If it isn't in biological balance, your body and your mind rebel.

When we make a drastic change, it's hard for our body and mind to stay with that change, so most of the time it wants to overcompensate for what's missing. This is the reason why when you think, "Ok, today I'm giving up chocolate completely," all you can think about is having 10 large chocolate bars. You might not have even thought about chocolate if you didn't declare such a drastic change. The Cheats and Eats Lifestyle Programme helps you make gradual, subtle changes so your body doesn't rebel. It makes small, good "deals" with your mind, so your body can get used to a new homeostasis. The Cheats and Eats Lifestyle Programme presents a new way of shedding pounds that your body says I can deal with this and you actually follow through. Whenever you embark on a lifestyle change that impacts your diet it's great to do as much reading as possible. It acts as reminder about why you're doing what you're doing and helps with that issue of follow through. I tend to use online resources like Healthspan (www. healthspan.co.uk) as an inspirational tool to learn about supplements, being active and well-being.

> The Cheats and Eats Lifestyle Programme is better than strict Paleo, where I could not eat beans or sweet potatoes.
>
> – Jessica

Just this Once...

The problem with restrictive diets is that it's really easy to fall off the wagon. And the second most people go the slightest bit off track, they use it as an excuse to go crazy for the rest of the day or even the rest of the week. You wake up on Monday morning and you want a fresh start...but then someone brings doughnuts to the office, or your car tyre is flat, or the buses are running late for work. So, you think, "Just this one morning I'm going to get my usual low-fat latte and a chocolate croissant, one last time." But by doing that, you set yourself up for a terrible lunch and dinner. You go out for Chinese with your co-workers for lunch and by dinner you figure it doesn't really matter so Monday is a total loss. So, then you decide, "I'm going to start Tuesday." And then Tuesday might go Ok, but when you weigh yourself on Wednesday it still isn't be better and you've been doing this all week and you decide that it doesn't matter what you do. And you give up once again.

You're probably very successful at other areas of your life. Why has weight loss been such a struggle? Here's why: in other areas of your life, you probably don't set unrealistic goals. In other areas of your life, when surprises happen that you don't expect, you probably roll with it, or at least handle it as best you can. When you slip up or do something wrong, you might chastise yourself for a moment and then let it go. When life happens, you don't beat yourself up.

But when it comes to dieting…you do all of those things. You set unrealistic goals of sticking to a restrictive diet. When a surprise is tossed your way – like doughnuts in the office – you freak out. When you eat a doughnut and slip up, you beat yourself up and decide that all your previous effort was a waste. This thought process is one of the biggest reasons other diets have failed you.

The fact is, diets stress people out. Workouts stress people out. Life stresses people out. And all those things are getting in the way of you losing the weight. From our experience and insight from people who have followed The Cheats and Eats Lifestyle Programme, we've found, overwhelmingly, that the pounds come off when the plan is easy, when it's doable and when it doesn't stress you out.

Stress Belly

Have you ever been ravenous *all* day? You get up hungry, eat your "normal" breakfast, and feel like in order to be full, you literally need to eat three more. Perhaps you've eaten two eggs, spinach and fruit, but you could eat another two plates of food and you're wanting a doughnut or something more than usual?

That may be cortisol at work and it could be one of the reasons you haven't been able to lose the weight or have that belly that you just cannot shift. A snacky, can't-get-full feeling may be cortisol out of balance. It's obvious why this is bad: if you're never full, then you're always eating, and that will definitely not help you lose weight.

This is a relatively new area of research investigating the link between stress, cortisol and the impact this has on weight. The effects of stress are particularly relevant to our modern fast-paced lifestyles, which can wreak havoc on our body and mind in many ways and is something that cannot be ignored. We're not saying cortisol is the sole reason people can't lose weight and the physiology is not that straight forward but this could be something that may be standing in the way for some of you. When we designed The Cheats and Eats Lifestyle Programme, this is one of the areas we took into consideration so that the foods you eat and the exercise you choose to do will work together to help combat the effects of this 'stress-hormone'.

Cortisol is a hormone released during events such as waking up, exercising and acute stress. It regulates energy by choosing the required amount of either carbohydrate, protein or fat depending on what the body needs. You may have heard of the 'fight or flight' response. This occurs when you are faced with a stressful event. Cortisol is released and floods the body with glucose (the simplest form of carbohydrate and preferred energy source) to give muscles an immediate supply of energy. Insulin (the hormone that reduces blood sugar) is also staved to prevent the glucose being stored and freely available to give you the immediate energy to deal with the event. Once the stress is addressed, hormone levels return to normal.

So, where's the problem? Issues may occur when we are exposed to chronic stress, which is a symptom of many people's modern lifestyles. A little stress is good and can give you the drive and energy you need to get through a job interview, work presentation or exam. More prolonged stress can occur when there is the constant worry caused by issues such as a high workload, job security, difficult relationship, bereavement and financial issues. You may feel overwhelmed, constantly 'wound up', constantly tired, anxious or depressed and find it difficult to concentrate or make decisions, lack self-esteem and have difficulty sleeping.

Research has shown how stress can impact on your immune system, raise blood pressure and increase your risk of heart disease and may cause you to gain weight[1]. Many people turn to unhealthy ways of trying to manage their stress such as drinking, smoking or comfort eating that can all affect your weight. Long-term stress results in a steady supply of cortisol that may be an underlying, physiological reason why you have difficulty losing weight. Chronic stress as well as a poor diet and being overweight can also increase inflammation (more on this later), which can further exacerbate the problem and impact on your long-term health.

Raised cortisol levels have been linked to weight gain[2] and a study carried out by researchers at the University College London found that people who had higher levels of this hormone in their body tended to have larger waist measurements and a higher body mass index[3].

Chronic stress has long been theorised as to be implicated with overweight and obesity in several ways. Firstly, cortisol can release fat from storage and transfer it to your belly, which in itself may also increase the production of this hormone. Secondly, high blood glucose teamed with insulin suppression (effect of cortisol) can starve cells of energy. The body responds by sending hunger signals to the brain, which may lead to overeating. In this case, any unused glucose will get stored as fat in the body. Thirdly, cortisol may affect appetite and cravings as demonstrated in a study published in the journal, *Psychoneuroendocrinology* that showed an association between raised cortisol levels and calorie intake in populations of women[4].

Interesting stuff but what has this got to do with The Cheats and Eats Lifestyle Programme? As we said earlier, cortisol may be one of the reasons dieting hasn't worked for you in the past so we made this a consideration when developing The Cheats and Eats Lifestyle Programme, reducing cortisol at every level: in the food you eat, when you work out, when and how often you feel stressed.

Learning how to manage your stress is key and if you think you are suffering with chronic stress then it is important you seek help from a qualified health professional. Food can play a part, especially with helping you to balance cortisol levels. Inflammation is linked to raised cortisol levels so The Cheats and Eats Lifestyle Programme encourages you to eat less inflammatory foods whist loading up on those that reduce inflammation and at the same time target cortisol. Exercise and practising some simple breathing techniques can also help and you will find more information about this in section three from leading UK personal trainer and wellness expert, Nicola Addison.

When you're eating the Eats from The Cheats and Eats Lifestyle Programme, Eats attack high cortisol head-on – which really helps to move the needle in the right direction when it comes to weight loss.

This is one of the major ways The Cheats and Eats Lifestyle Programme is different from any other diet you've tried: *It has taken into consideration the possible effects of cortisol and works to rebalance this hormone as well as other things that could be holding you back without you having to even think about it.*

Nice or Necessary?

Have you ever heard the story of the frog in warm water? If you put a frog in boiling water, he'll jump out. Instead, if you warm the water slowly, he will slowly die. You've got to create the "boiling" water in your life. You've got to create leverage. You've got to create your "must." Most of us say, "I want to lose a stone," but it doesn't really happen until we get focused and have the leverage like an event where we feel like we **must** do it. A school reunion is a good example. Many of us gain the leverage to lose weight when we know we're going to see peers from 20 years ago. The pain of not showing everyone what we could have been is *greater* than the pain of limiting Cheats and focusing on the Eats. So, we do it. Sadly, it often takes a diagnosis or a poor visit at the GP for many people to change their behaviours and make healthier lifestyle and diet choices. The positive here is that you finally have the leverage to change your habits.

So where do you get the *must* from? As you saw above, it usually comes from having a great need or the thought of extreme pain if you don't do something. The pain of facing people from secondary school at your current weight, and/or looking fat in the pictures on Facebook would have been greater than anything else happening before that weekend. Actors have they're must. They're always thin; they won't get paid if they are not. And pain – seeing a picture of yourself, hiding from social interaction – is sometimes what pushes people to lose weight. Another powerful must is being faced with a condition that can seriously impact on their quality of life such as diabetes.

I've heard a lot of desperation and frustration from people that email me and I've also seen how much creating and deciding upon your *must* can change your mind-set. Define your *need* to lose the weight. Define your why – *why* you want to lose the weight. Manufacture your *must* and change the game – putting you solidly on the path to success. You have nothing to lose but the weight that's been holding you back.

What's In Your Way (Other Than the Weight?)

When I'm eating and working out The Cheats and Eats Lifestyle Programme way, I know I'm going to lose weight. I'm confident of the end result. We will help you get confident, too. Losing weight on Cheat Lifestyle Programme will be so much easier than your path has been up to this point.

I suspect that having read the above, you are thinking, "You think weight loss is easy? You so don't know me, or my life, or what I'm going through!" But bear with me. When you obsess about something – whether it's about searching for the perfect relationship or worrying about how your child is going to get through school – you get in the way of the ease and flow that needs to happen in order for you to be successful. The best advice I've ever heard about dating is that when you want to fall in love, you shouldn't obsess over every phone call. You should make yourself busy, have your own interests, and then love will happen. The same applies to children: when you care about your kids but don't obsess over how every little thing in life is going to affect them, your children learn to stand on their own.

 I really like The Cheats and Eats Lifestyle Programme because it provides me an easy way to be accountable without being obsessive. It focuses on adding healthy foods that are beneficial to most people, yet gives you flexibility to make it your own.   – Eileen

The same applies to weight loss. Your obsession with weight loss is what's keeping you fat. I believe this with every fibre of my being.

It is the ease and the flow that allows the right date to become a permanent relationship, and allows parenting to transform a child into a functional adult. You're going to use the same principles with The Cheats and Eats Lifestyle Programme. It will give you ease and flow so you are not obsessed and beating yourself up the next time a brownie is calling your name. The Cheats and Eats Lifestyle Programme is about fitting into your life and getting rid of obsessiveness about losing weight.

Now you might be thinking, "Oh, they're just telling me to be positive, be positive, be positive." I'm not saying you should ignore the difficulty, and just pretend everything is Ok. Your frustrations are real and they are sabotaging you every day. It's about acknowledging them and moving on. The American life coach and philanthropist, Anthony Robbins often uses this really nice analogy in his talks: "I'm not telling you to look out in the garden and say there are no weeds. I'm telling you to look out in the garden, see the weeds and not say, 'Oh no, why are there weeds, why is this happening to me?' Instead, you'll go pull the weeds out and move on." That is what this book, and The Cheats and Eats Lifestyle Programme, will help you do.

We're going to pull out your weeds. And the first one I want to tug on is the belief that you have to do crazy things to lose weight. People have the idea that in order to lose weight, you have to eat lettuce and salads all day long, or foods you don't like, and oh, on top of that you have to work out hard for at least an hour every day, drink eight glasses of water, walk for four miles in the right shoes, and oh, P.S. you have to find a babysitter because you can't bring your kids and you need to find the money to pay for the gym and the right workout clothes, or a trainer…

When we think like this – and most of us do – we create what Dr. Pillay calls "brain chaos." Brain chaos is when there are so many signals and circuits lighting up in the brain that it can't make a decision. When the brain is experiencing chaos, we either do nothing about the situation, or we stress out by trying to do *everything*. When we encounter brain chaos as related to dieting, we either give up completely – "what's the use?" – or we try to incorporate everything we've ever heard, which also results in quitting.

It's insanity to expect success when you are putting too much pressure on yourself to do everything at once or when you give up completely. Neither is a clear path to your goal. However, when you ask your brain to do things that are easy for it to handle, you avoid brain chaos. We've created The Cheats and Eats Lifestyle Programme to do just that. It presents a set of rules that your brain can deal with, and doesn't ask you to do everything all at once.

What Do You, Personally, *Need* to Lose Weight?

Your answer to this question might be: *I have to have a babysitter. Or, I need a completely different way home from work, because the commute is long and I don't feel like eating healthy when I get home.* Whatever your need is, it's real and it's valid. You are smart, you are ambitious, you know what you want and in order to succeed, we need to harness those talents and to figure out how to make these obstacles to not losing weight disappear (or at least, get out of your way).

If you can identify your "if only" statement(s) for not losing weight – "if only I had money for a personal chef," or "if only I had money for a personal trainer," or "if only I wasn't so busy I could get to the supermarket to get healthy food" – you'll start to see something very interesting. We all have *if only* thoughts and the secret is, once you take care of one *if only*, a new one pops up.

The thing about *if only* is this: we believe that it's our "magic bullet" to losing weight. We believe it is the one thing holding us back from success. We all have *if only* reasons but the reality is that to lose weight, **dealing with where you are right now** is the magic bullet. This doesn't mean you shouldn't have wants and desires – you should, and I expect you to – but getting out of your own way (and making your *if only* reason disappear) starts with accepting and tackling the right now.

The first step to fulfilling your dream is accepting, right now, what your situation is. Right now, I don't have more money, I don't have a personal chef, I don't have a babysitter. But, given all of that, what *can* you do, or change, or try right now?

Eating well doesn't have to be expensive. You can train at home or walk to work. You don't need a trainer or expensive gym gear. Even if you could find a solution to your "if only", you may find that it still doesn't create a change. Once you accept this and start making real achievable changes that fit into everyday life you will start to get results.

Because You *Can* Lose Weight. And You *Will*

Get ready for a sentence that will change your life. If you're reading this in public place, go to a toilet or your car because I want you to say this life-changing miracle of a sentence with me. Say this out loud:

I am so frustrated with trying to lose weight. I'm so x%$@* frustrated!!!!
Say it a few times if it makes you feel better. See if it stops you from jumping on the stress treadmill where you constantly beat yourself up for being the size you are, eating the lunch you ate, drinking the wine you drank last night – you see where I'm going. Acknowledge what held you back and what's standing in your way now from losing the weight you want to lose. Now I'll begin giving you the tools with The Cheats and Eats Lifestyle Programme that will make weight loss seem doable – because you'll see results.

Why This Will Work (When Every Other Diet Hasn't)

If you haven't noticed already, the secret to The Cheats and Eats Lifestyle Programme's success is that we don't just tackle food and exercise. We know, from insight, that successful weight loss isn't just getting the food and exercise right, it's about the psychology: believing that you can do it and matching your desires to your expectations.

But The Cheats and Eats Lifestyle Programme attacks all the aspects holding you back from weight loss. Almost everything you

The Cheats and Eats Lifestyle Programme has been the *only* healthy eating plan that has ever worked for me! Not only has it enabled me to lose weight I never thought I would get rid of, it was so simple and it worked from the first day.

Please don't think it's just another diet; it isn't – it gets rid of cravings and it's simple and easy to follow. Please, please, give it a go – you won't regret it. After years of trying every diet out there, this was the answer to my prayers because it works!

– Dawn G

read in these pages will sound counter intuitive. For example, in this chapter, we talked about how to get your mind set on success, rather than focusing on dieting and repeating the same expectation of failure. In Chapter 2, we'll explain how you don't have to worry about fat content or fibre. In Chapter 3, with the help of Nicola, we'll discuss how you can start to workout in a way that doesn't stress you out. We'll help you to find your base so you can achieve something that is truly sustainable.

And in Chapter 4, we'll show you how you can eat whatever you want (within reason) – all of which will help you lose the weight that you've been trying to get rid of.

Yes, we're going to give you the plan. And yes, we're going to give you tips and tricks and advice and directions. And yes, we're going to give you the Cheat Sheet – Cheats And Eats – which is the key to The Cheats and Eats Lifestyle Programme. The Cheat Sheet breaks down every food, spice, herb, and beverage out there into two categories: the Eats – of which you can eat as much as you want – and the Cheats – which you limit but don't have to eliminate from your diet, ever.

I like the idea that nothing is truly off limits. I have a vicious sweet tooth and I'm a big carb addict. While I know carbs/sugar are the key to my weight gain, I know I can't just walk away from them and be happy. I like the idea that I can still acknowledge them as part of my diet.

Just do The Cheats and Eats Lifestyle Programme. It's probably the easiest "plan" I've ever seen. You can slowly add more and more healthy foods to your diet and slowly phase out the "cheats," at your own pace. I have *never* been successful for more than a couple days (if that) on a rigid system. I don't even bother with them. But this worked.

– Dawn M

You won't be white-knuckling it on this diet. There are more Eats that you can have unlimited portions of than there are Cheats. You won't be hungry, and you'll have plenty of energy to make good decisions and to keep making them.

How to Make this Programme Work for You

Four things to keep in mind as you start The Cheats and Eats Lifestyle Programme:

1. It's critical to have a road map.

No matter how much you commit to doing the diet, you are going to encounter pitfalls, setbacks and challenges. It is just a part of life. If you aren't prepared to deal with any of those things, though, then you'll find yourself dead in the water. There is always going to be temptation around you. There is always going to be the after-work socials, weekends away, birthday parties or cakes and biscuits brought in to work by your colleagues.

So, you have to have a road map that keeps you focused and on track when those temptations abound. You want to be able to enjoy them from time to time without going off the deep end. You have to have a way to build these types of events into your normal lifestyle or you will find yourself continually frustrated.

The Cheats and Eats Lifestyle Programme gives you that road map. It'll show you a simple way to keep track of your consumption without having to deprive and starve yourself.

2. Willpower is not enough.

Relying on your own willpower or discipline, as we discussed earlier, isn't a realistic or effective long-term weight-loss strategy. It is almost always a story with an unhappy ending. If you're white-knuckling your eating, the tension will eventually become too much and you will overeat.

When you're hungry – which you are when you are on a highly restrictive diet – you simply can't be disciplined or have willpower. Your stress and your hunger and your hormones overwhelm your body.

In order to succeed, you need to be well fed and happy – which is what The Cheats and Eats Lifestyle Programme does. When you deprive yourself, food is always on your mind. When you categorise foods as good and bad you see the odd treat as complete failure. But when you're well fed with healthy, high-nutrient foods and don't exclude the foods you enjoy eating, you're not thinking about food. You're just living your life, and that's a good thing. That's where we will be taking you.

3. Be patient and persistent.

You have to break the cycle of beating yourself up. You will be successful, but it's going to require some patience and persistence. You can't start eating the Eats and two days later be discouraged and give up if the scale doesn't move. All that does is further cement you in the faulty belief that it's not possible for you. Rubbish.

You *can* do this, but you have to be smart about it. It's not an overnight process (nothing that gives you real and lasting results is). It may take a bit of time to build the habits you need to get you there so take a deep breath...and now another...and one more...and smile and be easy on yourself. You need to treat yourself with at least compassion and understanding. Be easy on yourself and you'll get much further much quicker.

4. You don't have to be perfect to succeed, either.
As my great friend and American diet expert, JJ Virgin always says, "Go for the B+ not the A+." Perfection is impossible, and so is being 100 per cent on your diet all the time. But what *is* possible is being on the diet and doing what you should, eating what you should about 80 to 85 per cent of the time: the B+. We have built imperfection into The Cheats and Eats Lifestyle Programme – we are all human, after all! And even without perfection, it really works.

The whole idea of cheating allowed me to succeed without being perfect. Don't get it into your head that it is impossible; instead, see that it can and will work if you make wise choices and stick with them...

– Tom S

Before we get into the details of the diet in the next chapter, I understand that we've thrown a lot at you. We've explained how your brain works, We've explained that you need your *must*, and we will get into all of that later but right now, I want you to just think about one thing that's tripping you up. I know you're probably thinking, there are 150! But concentrate on one thing.

Is it the biscuits on your colleague's desk at work? Is it the play date where the other mums are drinking Chardonnay and you can't say no? Or is it date night? Or is it the fact that your husband or room-mate can eat whatever they want and not gain weight?

I want you to pick that one thing and I want you to give it up or avoid that habit for one day. You give up the biscuits in the office, or say no to the other mum's, or suggest an at-home date night where you make your husband or room-mate a healthy meal.

You will see the effect of making one small change. It's the accumulation of small changes that get results not matter how small they may seem. Before you start The Cheats and Eats Lifestyle Programme, you have to know that what you do will have a result and that you believe you can do it. We all still have a carrot-and-stick mentality, so you want and need your brain to be on board. Your brain must think that the changes you're making are a better deal. And you have to figure out what your *must* is. Write it down and write down your goal now. Make the water boil and jump out. And jump in to your new life.

CHAPTER 2

·

Why You Lose When You Cheat and Eat

If you're not taking care of you, you're not in a position to help anyone else. You can't give what you don't have...

– STEVE SIEBOLD

Maybe you wake up, excited to start your new morning regimen: egg whites, wholegrain bread, just a bit of low-fat cream cheese for breakfast, and you diligently head to the gym and hit the treadmill for 45 minutes – *every* day, all week. You make that yummy new wholewheat pizza recipe (it's wholegrain so you know it's good for you). You only go to lunch with your co-workers and eat "bad" food twice this week and maybe one night you couldn't stop eating the cheese and crackers. You think you've done your best but then you get on the scale you see not an ounce lost – or maybe you've even gained half of a pound. *Arggh.*

Or maybe you're the kind of person who reads all the latest health research, loves to make healthy recipes for your family and basically consider yourself a nutrition expert at this point. You have an incredible smoothie you drink for breakfast that contains two bananas, chia seeds, half an avocado, cacao nips, almonds, vegan protein powder, fibre and a whole bag of spinach. Your diet is all healthy right through dinner, with loads of seeds, nuts, beans, all vegan, everything the shows and the articles say will help you lose weight. So, you just don't get why the scale goes up one pound, down one pound, stays the same. All that work – and you're still a stone heavier than where you want to be.

Or you've just said to yourself: "I'm not going to diet. I can eat as long as I work out." And though you don't make a change nutritionally (well, maybe you have a bit less of this and a little more of that, because you're burning more calories now, and need more carbs or protein or whatever), you are a madman at the gym. One night, you can't resist a cheeseburger and a coke after a hard day and a long workout. You figure, "It can't do that much damage," but when you get on the scale the next day, your weight has gone up. Again.

Or maybe none of these scenarios rings true. You know what to do, and feel like you have a great deal of knowledge about how to lose weight and follow through, but you're just not doing it. You just don't feel like it. The motivation just isn't there. You feel like you'll have motivation again, someday – but not today. Not this month, and maybe not even this year.

Diet Confusion: Why You Can't Lose Weight Now

Whether you identified with one of the earlier examples or not, we all know that there are a million "right" diets that promise to work, and we all know – unfortunately, through experience – that most simply don't.

There is a huge and broad spectrum of diets out there for people to try. At one end, you have what we call the "traditional diet narrative": eating "healthy" foods like egg whites, wholegrains, and low-fat mayo with tinned tuna. That kind of diet really emphasises portion control and requires a lot of discipline and willpower. And though it can work in your twenties, when you're still the perfect hormonal specimen and may be able to resist the second slice of pizza, it may be more difficult after 35, when commitments become more of a barrier or your hormones have a greater impact. Some of us even find it difficult to stick to a portion-control diet even at a younger age.

At the other end of the spectrum you have more radical diets that encourage eating only raw vegetables or eliminating many foods. The research linking increased micronutrient intake to health states and weight loss is overwhelming and sure, vegetables do provide a rich source. No doctor will ever discourage an increase in eating vegetables.

And many physicians agree that the elimination of certain foods has proven to decrease inflammation and to have positive benefits. However, people find the vegetable-only plans and the elimination-of-entire-food-group plans challenging because the diet seems very restrictive and if you love food and approach it with a "live to eat" ethos, surviving on raw food is simply not going to work long term. Most don't know where to start and even those that do, end up finding these diets nearly impossible to follow through on.

It's important to note that all of these diets do "work" – but only if you can stick with them. If you are accurate at portion control, and can restrict your calories day in and day out, you can lose weight and maintain your weight loss. If you eat an entirely vegetable diet day in, day out, you will massively improve your health and you will lose the weight. If you permanently eliminate large categories of foods on an elimination diet, your inflammation will go down, and you will likely lose weight. However, these are often unsustainable and come with their own list of issues related to cutting out food groups, which over time can leave you at risk of nutrient deficiency if they are not followed properly.

From experience of observing thousands of people, we have come the conclusion that weight loss on these diets tends to be temporary. Because who can eliminate large food groups – wheat, eggs, dairy, corn, sugar, peanut butter – every day for the rest of their lives? We've seen that though many people can do this for a period of time (though some people can't do it at all) most fail at maintaining such a strict regimen.

If you want to lose weight and keep it off, you must marry what is scientifically proven to work for weight loss with what is doable in your life right now. And that's The Cheats and Eats Lifestyle Programme.

In creating The Cheats and Eats Lifestyle Programme, we reverse-engineered our diet plan. We knew a diet could work but that most people couldn't follow through. What we realised is this: the best information is recommended out of context. It doesn't take into consideration that we travel, that sometimes the only option is a ready-made meal or a fast-food restaurant. So, we started with a new question: What would people actually do, day in and day out, in real life?

The Three Essential Pillars

There are three major pillars that put the best, most up-to-date and proven science of weight-loss information into the context of everyday life – marrying what works with what's actually doable.

1. High-Nutrient Eating.
Eating foods with a high density of micronutrients – such as green leafy vegetables, beans and pulses – as well as protein, healthy fats and fibre is the key to feeling full and improving health.

2. Limiting Cheats.
The ability to eat foods you still want, need and crave – but keeping these foods a small part of your diet. A successful plan has to be flexible and forgiving enough to include social events where you'll have wine and dessert (and clear enough so that you understand exactly what and how much you are eating).

3. Reducing Cortisol and Inflammation.
The stress hormone cortisol and the inflammatory reaction from our immune system can work together and in some people this may make it difficult to lose weight as well as putting their health at risk further down the line. Eating the foods that help to reduce cortisol and inflammation may prevent your body from storing fat and assist in helping you to lose weight.

Cheat Lifestyle Programme Pillar #1: High-Nutrient Eating

Micronutrients. Beans. Vegetables. Have your eyes glazed over yet? Wake up! *Wake up!!* It isn't enough for you to eat your vegetables because everyone tells you to. You need to really know why you must eat them and the reasons have to be compelling – and they will be. In the UK, very few people manage to even eat five servings of fruits and vegetables, which is a long way off the updated recommendation of 10. As far as beans and pulses are concerned, they fail to make it to most people's plate.

I have a question for you to consider. Why can't we stop at one slice of pizza? Why is portion control so hard? *Because you can't control portion control when you are hungry.* Your hunger almost always takes over. You go in with good intent, thinking, "I'll just have one slice of cheese." Sometimes you can actually stop at one when you're focused, or when you have an event coming up and you have to lose the weight. But in real life, in everyday life? One slice becomes five – especially at night, or after you've had a bad day. The reality is, after one piece of pizza, you're actually still hungry – for good reason. The typical portion-control strategies set you up to eat a restricted amount of very low-quality nutrient foods. One piece of pizza rarely fills you up because there are very few good-quality nutrients in pizza, and only foods with a high-nutrient profile can curb your hunger. And this is because the only thing that makes you feel full is high-nutrient eating.

Micronutrients Versus Macronutrients

All food has macronutrients that are carbohydrates, fats and proteins. Carbohydrates and fats provide calories that in turn provide the body with energy. The most desirable energy source in the body is glucose that is derived from the breakdown of carbohydrates. While fats are used as the body's way of storing energy in the form of triglycerides.

Micronutrients include vitamins and minerals that are required to perform the physiological processes in the body that sustain life. A low intake of certain micronutrients can impact on energy in several ways. Iron for example (the most common deficiency worldwide), can inhibit the production of red blood cells that carry oxygen around the body and this increases the risk of anaemia, which flatlines your energy levels. B vitamins and magnesium on the other hand are required to convert macronutrients into energy at a cellular level and can cause tiredness and fatigue when you don't get an adequate intake of them.

Phytonutrients are compounds found in plants that are not essential for life but do help to protect the body from disease. The coloured pigments in plants are phytonutrients and include beta carotene found in orange and green fruits and vegetables or anthocyanins found in blue and purple fruits and vegetables. These share a common function as antioxidants and have been shown to reduce the risk of heart disease and cancer.

The micronutrient composition of foods varies widely. Sugar contains none and others such as broccoli contain lots. It's important to fill your diet with micronutrient-rich foods in a wide range of colours to get everything your body needs and dosing up on vegetables and other plant-based foods such as beans and pulses is the best way to do this. A diet rich in highly processed foods or sugar is not going to be as micronutrient-rich as a diet filled with foods that are eaten in their most natural state, which is why we encourage you to eat the Eats and limit your Cheats to achieve a happy medium.

On The Cheats and Eats Lifestyle Programme, you won't have to worry about any kind of nutrient because the diet does the hard work for you. We encourage lots of Eats because micronutrient-rich foods will not only ensure high energy levels but will also keep your body working at its optimum capacity. These foods are almost always high in fibre and that means keeping you full, which works with healthy fats and proteins for maximum effect.

The Best Diet Pill You Can Buy – At the Supermarket

If we were to put a hundred doctors and diet experts in a room, everyone would disagree about the best way to lose weight. But the one thing all those experts would agree with is that eating vegetables and other plant-foods such as beans and pulses is very important. Incorporating more of these foods in your diet will help you drop pounds, increase your energy and improve your overall health.

The concept is based around energy density. Low-energy density foods are high in water and contain a rich source of micronutrients but are low in calories. High energy density foods such as fried foods, fatty cuts of meats and high-fat dairy products contain more calories so less can be eaten and that also means less micronutrients. Low-energy density foods include vegetables, fruits, beans, pulses and lean cuts of meat rich in protein. You can combine these foods into dishes such as soups and stock, or tomato-based stews and other dishes to create low-energy density meals. The best thing about eating this way is that you can eat more food but still lose weight, which has been proven by scientific research[5].

Vegetables are a *must.* Most people know veggies are good for them nutritionally, but often don't include them in their meals with an after-thought of, "I'll do it next time." But here's the truth – research has shown that simply increasing the amount of high-nutrient food in your diet is *more effective* for weight loss than controlling or decreasing portion sizes of any food. In fact, people who eat high-nutrient foods not only tend to weigh less than people who eat more low-nutrient foods, **but they also eat more food.** You read that right. They eat bags more food, but they weigh less. You may be thinking, how is that possible?

There are three reasons why:

1. All Calories Are Not Created Equal

Keep in mind that 100 calories of salad are totally different than eating 100 calories of an apple, crisps or a chocolate bar. But here's what I want you to focus on, which comes back to the reason it's so hard to stop at one slice of pizza – if you choose the salad, you'll eat more food – and you'll be full longer.

Low-energy density foods are high in micronutrients and contain more fibre and water. Eating 100 calories of peppers, cucumbers, or spinach will make you feel fuller, for longer, than 100 calories of pasta or rice. Research has shown how foods with a higher water content can help keep you feeling full and assist with weight loss.

Our stomach digest foods with fibre slower than it digests anything processed. Your stomach digests a tablespoon of sugar in six minutes, whereas vegetables take an hour and pulses up to three hours, which means fuller for longer.

Before I Go On to #2...

I know what you're thinking: I'm telling you that eating vegetables is going to help you lose weight – and you're probably just thinking: I've heard this before! But I promise you, vegetables are going to be your new best friend. When you focus on Eats such as artichokes, salsa and sweet potatoes, you'll not only be fuller for longer and have tons of energy but you'll make better decisions – all of which combines into weight loss.

Let me show you a simple diagram of three stomachs, used with permission from Dr. Joel Fuhrman's book *Eat to Live*. With over 1,200 references supporting high-nutrient foods and health, *Eat to Live* is the most well-structured argument out there for why vegetables are king for weight loss. The following diagram shows what your stomach looks like when it eats 400 calories each of fat (an oil), a protein (chicken), and Eats. (Joel used spinach, aubergine and beans.)

MORE BULK MEANS FEWER CALORIES

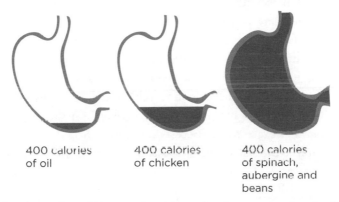

400 calories
of oil

400 calories
of chicken

400 calories
of spinach,
aubergine and
beans

Look at that! No wonder it's so hard to maintain the high-protein-and-nothing-else diets. Your stomach needs foooooood. It needs micronutrients. It wants to feel full. It doesn't care about "nothing tastes as good as thin feels" – because thin doesn't feel good.

2. The Best Little Fat Burners In The World

On The Cheats and Eats Lifestyle Programme, you can eat however much it takes of the Eats – which are all high micronutrient foods – that you need to feel satiated and full. You can eat as much as you want, no restrictions, because Eats are the key to you feeling full. How did we discover this "full" secret while everyone else is out there chanting willpower slogans while they're starving? After we met Dr. Joel Fuhrman, and then read his books and research, it was impossible to go back. In *Eat to Live*, he proves that even if you eat more volume (a bigger amount) of low-energy dense, high micronutrient foods than you would of high-energy dense, low micronutrient food, you end up eating fewer calories. Fuhrman's programme is based on the acronym G-BOMBS (greens, beans, onions, mushrooms, berries and seeds) the highest level of micronutrients. Consider kale (or spinach, or greens) versus rice. One hundred calories of cooked kale is about 350g, whereas 100 calories of cooked rice is only 75g. (If you were to eat 100 calories of pizza, that would be half a typical slice.) You may have eaten the same number of calories, but the kale gives you more bang for your buck – and you will feel full!

And here is where it gets interesting: Eats not only keep you feeling full, they help you burn fat. The Eats, especially mushrooms (always make sure they're cooked), function as "angiogenesis inhibitors". Angiogenesis is a process that results in the growth of new blood vessels from pre-existing vessels.

What's interesting is that the growth of fat tissue is dependent on this exact same process and researchers have begun to explore the role that angionesis may play in the prevention of obesity[6]. When you increase the amount of high-nutrient foods, especially broccoli, mushrooms, onions, greens and berries, you are eating a diet that fights angiogenesis, making it hard for fat to get its own blood supply and grow.

Researchers are starting to look into what they call "pharmacological manipulation of adipose [body fat] tissue [to] offer a novel therapeutic option for the treatment of obesity and related metabolic disorders." Translated that means that drug companies are trying to turn the properties of these foods into drugs. But you don't need that – you just need to eat the Eats in order to give your body the same results: losing weight.

3. No More Hunger or Toxic Withdrawal

I was with a relative a few months ago at lunchtime, and we both made salads for ourselves. I made a huge salad and filled a large bowl, similar in size to a family salad bowl. She made a salad about one-third the size of mine and placed it on a square appetiser-size dish. So, we ate: my salad in this huge bowl, and hers on this little dish. We had nearly identical salads but we had completely different portion sizes.

When we were, both done eating, she said that she was still hungry; she actually said, "I'm starving." I responded, "Of course you're still hungry! Who wouldn't be starving on that little tiny dish of salad?"

"You ate a pretty big bowl, didn't you?" she replied. I told her that I always eat out of a big family-sized bowl or order at least two or three vegetables sides at a restaurant, because that's what keeps me from being hungry.

She responded, "Do you think I could make and eat another salad and still lose weight?"

The answer is yes. YES! YES! YES! Vegetables are the best diet pill in the supermarket. I told her to go out that day and buy two *large* salad bowls. Why two? Because if you have two, then one will almost always be clean.

The truth is, most of us don't eat enough high-nutrient foods (Eats) to not feel hungry. But on The Cheats and Eats Lifestyle Programme, you will – your body will be getting what it needs to feel full and satiated, even between meals.

A study published in 2010 *Nutrition Journal*[7] showed how people who ate low-nutrient dense foods tended to be hungrier more often than people with high-nutrient dense diets. That may be why, when you eat a sandwich for lunch, you end up craving a latte and a scone just a few hours later.

Interestingly, the researchers hypothesised that one of the reasons why the people in the study had less hunger on a high-nutrient dense diet is because a low-nutrient dense diet can cause "toxic hunger," hunger that wasn't true hunger but rather was caused by metabolic dysfunction. Increasing nutrient density reduces the feeling of toxic hunger, making the sensation of hunger much more tolerable.

While eating a diet high in vegetables and fruits, your body simply doesn't have the same hormonal reactions as it would on a portion-controlled only diet. Your blood sugar and insulin are relatively stable and your body doesn't freak out about having enough food to fuel itself. You feel full, and because you're eating enough during the day, you don't dive into the cheese and crackers every night. That said, we still want to be able to have cheese and crackers. We can't only eat high-nutrient foods one hundred per cent of the time. Well most of us can't. Which is why The Cheats and Eats Lifestyle Programme works. You feel full of your Eats but you still have your Cheats. Like a glass of wine. Or chocolate. Or bacon. Or whatever you need to feel satisfied.

Are You "Good" All Day, But "Mess Up" at Night?

From listening to people who have followed are diet plan, we have seen a phenomenon where people feel as if they do great all day, and then "mess up" at night. We've figured out why this happens – and the solution is right here in this chapter. The reason that you find it impossible to resist the cheese in the fridge and the crackers in the cupboard is because you're not eating enough high micronutrient food during the day. This is why in The Cheats and Eats Lifestyle Programme; many foods are *unlimited*. If you're full at breakfast, lunch and dinner, you'll be able to say no to the cheese or chocolate at night – because your body will have had everything it needs for the day.

There is so much pushing against you from succeeding when you diet. Most of the time, you're not getting the emotional, physical, or nutritional support your body needs to operate at its best. But The Cheats and Eats Lifestyle Programme will provide your body with the physical and nutritional resources it needs to lose weight – and curb the late-night trips to the fridge that are holding you back now.

On The Cheats and Eats Lifestyle Programme you're going to feel full. Because you're going to be eating *unlimited* amounts of Eats. We're going to show you how to do it – you're not going to have to white-knuckle it through the evening anymore after a really hard day. And when you're at a party, you're still going to be able to eat cheese. You're still going to be able to have chocolate. That's where the second pillar comes in…

Cheat Lifestyle Programme Pillar #2: Limit Cheats

To make anything stick for the long term, you're going to have to be able to live in the "real world". You're going to have to be able to go to a party and not stress out about food. This is where the second pillar comes in – being able to eat foods you love, but with the plan of knowing your Cheats. When you know your Cheat limit, you can still have Cheats and lose weight. This is all about the delicious Cheats.

This is not about eliminating foods, or counting and figuring out every single calorie, fibre and fat, and measuring everything you eat because both of those things are untenable. There will always be a day you're stressed out and you go off track. You still have to eat at your mother-in-law's, your friends will still want to try the amazing new bakery and you will want a cupcake. But most important, if you try to do a portion-control-only diet, you'll almost always be wrong: you'll almost always be eating more than you think.

How does portion distortion happen? It can happen when you start to date someone new or get married, or when you see your partner eat a lot more than you. Suddenly, your idea of portions get skewed. Or maybe when you were pregnant your hormones went out of control and you ate everything in sight. And now you're post-pregnancy, and after nine months, it's hard to eyeball what a "reasonable" portion is anymore. And additionally, you find yourself obsessing about food all the time.

In a 1993 study published in the *New England Journal of Medicine*[8], which was later repeated and proven by similar studies, researchers asked participants to record their calories. The researchers then compared what the participants said they ate to what they actually ate. The participants under reported their daily average intake by 47 per cent! That would be the real-world equivalent of eating 147 calories, while thinking that you only ate 100. If you were following a calorie-counting or portion-control-only diet, at 1,700 calories in a day, you could be eating 799 more calories a day! That's almost 800 calories more – 2,500 calories a day in reality versus what you are thinking you're eating: a 1,700-calorie-a-day diet. And that's 3,500 more calories per week. You can just imagine what can happen after a month and a year. No wonder portion control fails so many people.

Why Portion Control Failure Is Not Your Fault

Even when people are taught accurate portions, they can't keep to their diet. In two different studies[9, 10], done years apart, researchers tested how well people gauge proper portions and each time, got the same result. In both studies, the researchers divided participants into four groups. Each group was taught proper portions: how much and what to eat. Three groups were given meals with correct portions measured for them and the fourth group had to make their own meal after just learning proper portions. I'm sure you can guess what happened. The groups who were given the meals lost more weight than the group who had to make the meal themselves. They were all taught proper portion control. They just couldn't do it on their own.

There's also a psychological component. In a different experiment[11], researchers asked participants to eat a bowl of soup that was supposedly the "right" portion size. But what the participants didn't know was that one bowl was "normal" and the other was bottomless.

When comparing the two groups after the study, researchers found that the people who had the bottomless bowl ate more. But here's the kicker: the people who ate out of the bottomless bowl didn't feel any more satiated than the group that had eaten the standard portion in the normal bowl. What the scientists concluded in that study was that perhaps visual cues – what size portions we see on our plate – affects our hunger and feeling full more than what we *actually* eat.

Portion control works, to some extent – which is why on The Cheats and Eats Lifestyle Programme, you'll count the Cheats you eat. Portion control is more successful if you have a lot of forgiveness built in. That's why we make it a part of The Cheats and Eats Lifestyle Programme. You can have bacon – one medium slice of cooked bacon is one Cheat – but you'll be coupling those calories with feeling full and lots of micronutrients, not depending on the bacon alone to fill you up. When you count your Cheats, and eat your Eats, you'll be able to lose weight and still go to a dinner party. And you can have some ice cream when you're really stressed. Because these Cheats are part of the plan – they won't destroy your entire weight-loss strategy.

Cheat Lifestyle Programme Pillar #3: Reducing Inflammation and Shrinking the Fat Storage System

In Chapter 1, we discussed how cortisol might be the reason you haven't been able to lose the weight. There are two other major biological factors that impact weight, both how much we lose and how much we gain: inflammation and hormones.

Inflammation: The Biggest Weight Loss Inhibitor

Inflammation is a reaction from our immune system. Given the amount of negative press it receives there is a misconception it's all bad but it's actually essential to life. Inflammation occurs in two forms referred to as acute and chronic.

Acute inflammation is obvious and more visible; you cut yourself, the body sends out an army of white blood cells and you experience the associated redness, heat and swelling. When the injury is healed, acute inflammation is gone. This type of inflammation also protects your body from foreign invaders that can threaten your health.

Chronic inflammation, on the other hand, can be pretty covert: it can be present in the body for a long time without being visible or noticeable. The immune system continues to respond to one or more factors that can include environmental toxins, stress and poor diet. It becomes uncontrolled as it fails to maintain homeostasis and the long-term result is a series of destructive reactions that damage cells and cause disease.

Being overweight is a key driver for chronic inflammation and is thought to be an adaptive response to overeating[12]. We now know that fat cells stored around your middle are not just a way to reserve energy but are metabolically very active and churn out hormones, proteins, growth factors and inflammatory cells that regulate your food intake and metabolism of fats and carbohydrates. As you gain more weight around your middle, the fat cells grow and change shape, which initiates an inflammatory response. The longer you are overweight, the longer this flame will keep burning throughout the body causing damage.

Inflammation may even play a role in weight gain as research has suggested that the process may influence the hormone leptin, that is involved in appetite regulation[13]. A large study published in the journal *Obesity* also found that inflammation acted as a predictor of future weight gain amongst overweight adults[14].

The hormone cortisol that we mentioned earlier can also increase inflammation in the body so eating the right diet to help you to reduce cortisol and reduce inflammation may not only help you to lose weight but protect your long-term health.

There is no doubt that an anti-inflammatory diet is going to be beneficial to your health and may even assist you to lose weight. The Mediterranean diet is often cited as being anti-inflammatory and on paper it is nothing you probably don't already know. Plenty of plant-based foods, good-quality protein and healthy fats. The Cheats and Eats Lifestyle Programme reflects this healthy way of eating and has done the hard work for you so you don't have to think about it.

The basics of anti-inflammatory eating involve:
+ A low glycemic load diet (plenty of protein, healthy fats and high fibre foods with less sugar and quickly digested carbohydrates)
+ Reduced caffeine
+ Reduced alcohol
+ Increased intake of whole plant foods such as vegetables that are nutrient rich including vitamins, minerals, phytonutrients and antioxidants
+ Plenty of omega-3 fatty acids and less omega-6 fatty acids to achieve a balance of these essential fats

Decreasing the inflammation in your body is the key to unlocking weight loss – because if you get rid of inflammation, you get rid of fat.

For any of you still under the impression that fat is bad, it's important to understand that we need some fat to survive and healthy fats are essential in the fight against inflammation. Fat in the diet doesn't necessarily make you fat. The key take home message here is that if you are overweight then you are encouraging inflammation. Losing weight means lowering inflammation, which means losing fat.

What Does Work: Diet *Fusion* (Not Confusion!)

Some diets work and some work up to a point. Portion control works for some, up to a point. The elimination diets reduce inflammation and help you lose weight but almost everyone trips up at a party or breaks down one night and binges on cheese, which means they are often unsustainable. Veganism is really popular at the moment and does help some people to lose weight, but the restrictiveness is often difficult to maintain outside of your own kitchen and when not followed properly can leave you lacking in essential nutrients.

What the diet world needs is something that takes the best ideas and brings them together in a plan that really works. This is exactly what The Cheats and Eats Lifestyle Programme does. We call this concept *diet fusion*, and it's the foundation of The Cheats and Eats Lifestyle Programme. We understand that nutrient-rich foods, including vegetables – what we call Eats – are king, while at the same time acknowledging that we live in the real world and are going to have a cookie or enjoy a cheese board at a party.

The Cheats and Eats Lifestyle Programme is common sense. You eat healthy most of the time, so it's Ok to indulge yourself every once in a while. You'll eat well 80 per cent of the time, so the other 20 per cent doesn't matter nearly as much as if you ate that food all the time.

On The Cheats and Eats Lifestyle Programme, you don't have to do any of that. You don't need to count calories or worry about macro and micronutrients because we've figured that for you. We've divided foods into two different categories: the Eats and the Cheats. This is the marriage between what works and what's actually doable, and it's what will help you lose the weight.

Why Cheating and Eating Works

The Cheats and Eats Lifestyle Programme has you eating the same way that studies have shown lower caloric intake overall, reduce hunger and cravings, and increase the level of satiety at every meal. While portion control has been shown over and over again in scientific studies *not* to work unless you are served pre-portioned meals in a controlled environment or plan to eat all pre-packaged meals, there have been studies that show how people who eat a **diet with a foundation similar to The Cheats and Eats Lifestyle Programme lose three times as much weight as people who rely on portion control alone.**

In fact, some of the most successful, clinically-studied diets, including one featured in the journal *Nutrition Reviews* in 2001[15], use the exact same approach as The Cheats and Eats Lifestyle Programme: eating foods that are good for your body with small amounts of Cheats.

Eat the Eats, but Count Your Cheats

The mistake many of us make when we're busy and just trying to get things done is that we don't think our food choices through. We think, "Oh, just this one time couldn't hurt." But it's never just one time. One time leads to another one time, and then it's multiple times, which end up stacking up into pounds gained. I remember the day I discovered the salted caramel hot chocolate at Starbucks. I said, "Ok, I'm just going to get a small." Well, I did that every day for a month.

One day, I thought, "What's really in this thing?" So, I asked. The barista started reading the ingredients and I couldn't believe what I was actually drinking! The signature drink was around three Cheats and that was without the whipped cream.

We are all going to make mistakes, including me. And you're probably going to make those mistakes more often than you like. But the best thing about Cheat Lifestyle Programme is that you're able to make mistakes. You don't need to be perfect because The Cheats and Eats Lifestyle Programme is designed for that. When you eat a truly healthy diet most of the time, eating Cheats won't harm you as much as it would a person who *only or mostly* eats those foods.

Cheating + Eating = Energy

Every meal on The Cheats and Eats Lifestyle Programme will provide you with enough energy to sustain you through the day. You may find that you feel more energy than you have in years. That's because a typical meal on The Cheats and Eats Lifestyle Programme has everything your body needs to function – without the rush/crash/rush cycle that sugar and caffeine have.

One of the most important lessons we learned is that you have to have energy to make good decisions, and that your weight loss really hinges on what kind of decisions you make. Most decisions that really affect weight loss seem simple: I'm going to have a salad with chicken at lunch, or I'm going to have the pasta. You simply choose the healthy choice or the not-healthy or less-healthy choice. With each decision, you are making a deal with your brain; for every small choice you make, your brain has to feel like you're making the better choice.

For instance, let's talk about French fries. Once you tell yourself you can never eat French fries, your brain goes "Wait, that's not a great deal!" – so it starts freaking out. However, since you can eat anything you want (including French fries) on The Cheats and Eats Lifestyle Programme, if you decide to pass on French fries at lunch, your brain says, "Oh, no problem, I can eat French fries another time. I can do that."

Drink Water!

Consuming water is the best, most important thing you can do for your body – and for weight loss. Our body is mostly composed of water – because nearly everything needs it, from cells in our organs to our blood and our brain. When you don't drink enough water, your body simply doesn't perform the way it should. Without enough water, your muscles may even be weaker, making any workout or physical activity you do less productive.

Try and drink at least eight glasses of water each day. If you don't like the taste of water for whatever reason, feel free to naturally flavour it with berries, grapefruit, lemon, or cucumber (which are Eats). Research published in the journal Obesity showed how drinking a glass of water before and after you eat may help assist with weight loss[16].

What Cheating and Eating Looks Like On a Plate

A Cheat Lifestyle Programme meal combines healthy fats, traditional protein and Eats to provide all the energy you need for the day. These three things should always be on your plate. I understand that I said "always," but this is ideal. If you can't, you can't — don't let that stress you out and drive up your cortisol.

1. Healthy Fats

Healthy fats are essential. Without them, you wouldn't be able to live. Healthy fats include omega-3 fatty acids (found in fish, fish oil, chia and flaxseeds) and mono-unsaturated fats (found in olive oil, nuts, seeds and avocados), all of which have positive benefits to health by reducing inflammation, thinning the blood and reducing bad cholesterol.

Fat is essential for health and current research has painted a much clearer picture of the role this macronutrient plays in the body. Current guidance is to focus on eating mostly 'good' fats in your diet. By doing this you will naturally be limiting the bad fats that can promote inflammation and contribute to your risk of heart disease and other conditions.

Healthy fats make us feel satiated and give meals a better taste and mouth feel. When you add a good fat to a meal, it will not only make the dish tastier but help to keep you feeling full between meals, which means less chance of snacking.

Omega-3 fatty acids are often referred to as being essential, which means they need to be obtained from your diet as the body can't make them. The most beneficial of these are EPA and DHA, found mostly in oily fish. If you don't eat oily fish then the body can make these two fatty acids from another type of omega-3, called ALA, which is found in walnuts, dark green leafy vegetables, nuts and seeds. The problem is that this conversion is very poor and whilst they are a useful source you should take a daily 1000mg omega-3 supplement that contains both EPA and DHA fatty acids.

By now you probably understand the importance of managing inflammation in your diet. Omega-6 fatty acids are essential to a healthy diet but when eaten in excess, these can also promote inflammation. Oily fish intake in the UK is low, with many people not eating a single portion on a weekly basis, meaning our intake of omega-6 often outweighs that of omega-3. Eating more oily fish or taking a supplement is key but cutting back on omega-6 can also be very beneficial. Switching to extra virgin olive oil as your main cooking fat alongside coconut oil, choosing butter over margarine, cutting back on your meat intake and choosing grass-fed, whilst also avoiding highly processed or take-away meals will have a big impact on this balance and help tackle inflammation.

Sugar and Fat

In the popular book by the author, Michael Moss, he shows how food scientists have worked very hard to create the right amount of sugar, salt and fat in processed foods so that people will keep eating. The right combination of these will create the satiation point: where the food is flavourful, but bland enough to keep eating – like the perfect potato chips. A meal that is greater or lower than this point will not have this same effect.

No physician or nutritionist will dispute that large amounts of sugar is bad. Most people know that eating sugar adds calories, and it does. But the bigger issue is that sugar can cause the same reactions in your brain as cocaine. Once you have some, you will always want more. That's why we consider processed and sugary foods "Cheats".

Food surveys in the UK show that we are all eating way too much sugar, which is reflected across the globe. Eating lots of sugar in the diet is now widely recognised as playing a very influential part in the obesity dilemma plaguing the world and is responsible for increasing inflammation in the body as well as your chances of developing a number of chronic diseases.

Sugar appears in many foods in one way shape or form. Cutting right down is key and something The Cheats and Eats Lifestyle Programme takes care of for you. To remove sugar completely from your diet is actually very tricky and generally not sustainable in the long-term, which is why there is some room in The Cheats and Eats Lifestyle Programme for a little bit of the sweet stuff.

Don't be fooled into thinking any of the so called 'healthy' sweeteners are any better than cane sugar. There is no such thing as a healthy sweetener. Whilst agave, honey, maple syrup, date syrup or coconut nectar may be a slightly better choice to cane sugar, there is no health benefit associated with these foods. They're not health foods. Sugar is sugar, whatever form it comes in.

When you eat a meal, your blood sugar will naturally rise and a hormone called insulin goes to work at lowering your blood sugar. But when you eat a meal or a snack or a drink containing a lot of sugar, your blood sugar can take a sudden spike. Your body will respond by releasing insulin to drive sugar out of the blood and to areas of the body that need it. Some glucose is stored in the muscles and liver as glycogen then anything left over is converted to triglycerides and stored in fat tissue. Insulin also inhibits the body from using fat for energy.

All carbohydrate foods are broken down into glucose but those that contain more fibre have less impact on blood sugar levels and hunger. Foods rich in quickly digested carbohydrates and especially sugar can give you a quick energy rush but more often than not this is quickly followed by a sugar crash that can leave you feeling lethargic and a victim of the mid-morning or mid-afternoon energy slump. If insulin does its job really well – which it typically does – you also end up feeling hungry again almost right away. When there is too much sugar in your diet, it's very, very easy to overeat, and not realise it. You can slow down this process by serving quickly digested carbohydrates such as white pasta and rice with healthy fats, proteins and vegetables (high in fibre).

There is a large body of research highlighting the negative impact that too much sugar can have on your health beyond weight gain. Table sugar is also known as sucrose, which is made up of glucose and fructose. The use of glucose in the body is strictly controlled by insulin, as we mentioned earlier. However, when the body has used the fructose it needs for energy the excess becomes part of a process that forms fatty acids in the liver, which are then transported as a harmful type of cholesterol known as Very Low Density Lipoproteins (VLDL). This type of cholesterol is easily oxidised and has been shown to be a major risk factor for heart disease.

Eats and Cheats is not a low carbohydrate diet, but these foods are controlled so you don't overeat them. Teamed with protein, healthy fats and high-fibre foods you will be able to control your blood sugar levels and increase satiety, which means less hunger pangs, cravings and energy slumps. By regulating the amount quickly digested carbohydrates in your diet, you will be providing your body with what it needs to match your energy requirements as well as burning more fat. This is another reason for sticking to three meals a day and cutting out snacking, which can impact on blood sugar fluctuations, encourage fat storage and provide you with another potential opportunity to overeat.

If this isn't enough to persuade you to cut down on your sugar intake then maybe vanity might encourage you. There is some evidence to suggest that excess sugar can promote skin ageing by accelerating a process called glycation that can increase skin stiffness and reduced elasticity[17]. It's not fully proven and the research is based on mice studies but many people who cut down on sugar notice a difference in their skin.

2. Traditional Animal Protein or Plant Protein?

Protein is essential to the diet as it helps to promote the growth and repair of tissues, makes hormones and can help to keep you feeling full. Protein is made up of amino acids, nine of which are essential and need to be obtained from the diet.

Animal proteins include meat, fish and eggs. These foods contain all of the essential amino acids that make up proteins (the building blocks). Plant sources of protein include quinoa, buckwheat, beans, peas, lentils, pulses, nuts and seeds. Some of these foods do not contain all of the essential amino acids but when they are included in meals across the day non-meat eaters will get all the amino acids they need as long as they are eating enough protein. The Cheats and Eats Lifestyle Programme promotes eating a source of protein with every meal.

Although most of us generally eat more than adequate amounts of protein in our diet, certain groups may not get enough. Non-meat eaters, mainly vegans, may not eat enough protein to promote weight loss. It's not impossible, and many vegans manage their diet very well, but it is difficult. Studies published in the *New England Journal of Medicine*, the *Journal of Cardiovascular Nursing*, and *Nutrition* have shown that diets eliminating animal proteins may not be as successful in dropping pounds. Supplementing your diet with protein powder can be a useful way to add this nutrient to your diet and support weight loss.

Drinking a breakfast smoothie made from plant-based protein kick-starts your day's fat burning by balancing blood sugar or insulin levels. A study in the *American Journal of Clinical Nutrition*[18] showed a high-protein breakfast reduced ghrelin – a hormone that tells your brain to eat – better than a high-carb breakfast did. Lower ghrelin, coupled with a balanced blood sugar level, mean you're far less likely to make that mid-morning biscuit tin raid or vending machine trip.

That's why, on Cheat System, we ask for you to eat 100g of traditional lean animal protein, such as chicken, fish, beef or an egg, or a serving of plant protein from a quality source with every meal. And like the healthy fat, 100g of traditional protein or one serving of plant protein at your first meal is also Cheat free!

Why Do We Advocate for Traditional Protein or Plant-Based Protein?

These kinds of protein will keep you satiated. If you were to eat large portions of vegetables without traditional or plant protein, you eventually would be satiated (remember those three stomachs). But most people don't eat enough vegetables to reach that point. You would have to eat two or three starter portions of salads and vegetables to reach that point, for a typical nine stone woman. Most people aren't willing to do that. Remember, I'm obsessed with follow-through and for many people, it's just too hard to eat enough vegetables, without traditional protein, to feel satiated. So, this is why we advocate a traditional protein.

What Kinds of Traditional Protein Should You Eat?

Beef: There are significant nutritional differences in your beef choice depending on how meat is raised. Grass-fed is always the better choice but we get that this is not always available. Conventionally-raised beef has much more fat than grass fed beef – almost two and half times as much! If you're thinking, "But I trim the fat off my steak anyway," and while that's great to do, it doesn't really solve the problem. Conventionally raised cattle mostly eat grain like corn, which results in their muscles being marbled and makes for a tasty steak, but because the fat is intertwined with the muscle, it is impossible to "trim" this kind of fat from a cut of meat.

Grass-fed beef also has more healthy fats (for example, omega-3s) than traditionally raised beef. Omega-3s are cheap calories: omega-3s are used for maintaining and building cell membranes. They don't get stored as fat. (The only people known by researchers to actually store significant amounts of omega-3 calories as fat are the Inuit, who eat a fish-based diet. They consume so many omega-3s, they are basically forced to store some, but even they only store about one per cent of what they eat.)

So, go grass-fed when you can, but don't stress about it. If you can't afford or find grass-fed beef, buy the leanest cut you can.

Try not to make beef your first choice of protein every day and limit the amount of processed meat (bacon, sausages and ham) you eat. We all love a bit of bacon but advice from the World Health Organization (WHO), based on the findings of scientific research[19] is that a diet rich in red meat and more so, processed meat is significantly associated with an increased risk of colorectal cancer. Limit your red meat intake to no more than five times per week (five, 100g servings) and treat sausages, bacon and ham as the occasional Eat rather than an everyday choice.

On another note, trying to go veggie for one day each week is a nice campaign to reduce the environmental damage caused by the farming of cattle to meet the world's demand for this food.

Chicken: Free-range chickens are better than conventional chickens that live in tight buildings . Conventional chickens are traditionally fed grains (making them high in omega-6) and antibiotics to grow bigger and survive the tough conditions. Additionally, conventionally raised chickens are loaded with chemicals and tend to have more unhealthy fats than organic, free range, or pasture-raised chicken. Free-range chickens are allowed to walk around outside and have a diet that combines natural grass and plants with their feed.

Organic chickens, the next step up, are free-range and have been raised in a natural environment – no antibiotics allowed. And pasture-raised, the best of all, means that the chickens are not only allowed to roam but eat only what they would in the wild, mostly seeds, weeds and bugs.

So, if you can, buy free range or pasture-raised eggs and chickens. You'll notice a difference in how they taste – and for eggs, even how they look. Factory-farm egg yolks are usually a light yellow, whereas free-range eggs and pasture-raised eggs are a much deeper yellow from the extra beta-carotene they contain.

Fish: When it comes to fish, wild is better. It's leaner and has more omega-3s as a percentage of total fat than farmed fish. Salmon is a great example: farmed salmon has much more fat than wild salmon. Farmed salmon has omega-3s, but also contains a lot of omega-6s (fats we should limit). Omega-3s and omega-6s both wind up in our cell membranes, and how much we eat of each one determines whether the healthy, anti-inflammatory omega-3s dominate or whether the inflammatory omega-6s dominate.

In farmed fish, there are loads of omega-6s that skew the balance; in wild fish, the omega-3s vastly outnumber the omega-6s. So, while eating a farmed fish would be better than a grain-fed steak or a factory-farm chicken breast, it's not nearly as healthy as wild fish.

Toxins are one of the main reasons that nutritionists don't advocate eating fish for every meal. If you focus on eating the smaller fish on the food chain such as salmon and haddock rather than the larger ones such as tuna and Chilean sea bass, you'll avoid the problems associated with the toxins in fish, such as mercury.

On The Cheats and Eats Lifestyle Programme, we'd love for you to try eating oily fish at least once a week. And be sure to take a daily 1000mg omega-3 supplement if you can't manage that.

What is the difference between protein powders?
Pea and Rice Protein. It's a complete protein, has the same amount of branched-chain amino acids as meat, and it's a great short cut for breakfast. It fills you up and the protein releases slowly. In fact, pea protein releases more slowly than the whey protein in most "energy" shakes, which makes you feel fuller, longer.

Is Whey or Soy Protein as Good as Pea and Rice or Pea and Potato Protein?

Pea and rice protein, when mixed together, form a complete protein (pea is low in sulfur-containing amino acids while rice is high). The sports nutritionist, Brian Rigby explains, "while whey and soy are also complete proteins, they have a high allergenic nature. Soy can cause sensitivities and inflammation and the soy protein isolate used in soy protein powder can also be higher in isoflavones than soy products which have not been processed and concentrated like soy protein isolate has been."

Whey can still be a trigger for sensitivities in certain people. Because whey protein is rapidly absorbed, most of it will end up as nitrogen waste in the urine unless you are a serious athlete and just going to or returning from exercise! Pea and rice protein, on the other hand, is digested and absorbed more slowly, causing it to be more satiating for people trying to lose weight and ensuring that the majority of it goes toward maintaining lean body mass, not getting excreted as waste.

Pea and rice protein is highly digestible and readily absorbed. If you are concerned about exercise and protein for recovery, pea and rice protein is comparably high in the branched-chain amino acids (BCAAs), arginine, and lysine as whey protein, making it equal in terms of muscle recovery, strength training and fat burning. When choosing a protein powder, look for one that is sugar free.

The Star of the Show: Unlimited Eats

Eat Your Eats – as much as you want, any time you want. Berries, cucumbers, grapefruit, artichokes, spinach, Swiss chard, asparagus, butternut squash, sweet potato fries, peppers, salsa, kale, mushrooms. There's no need to portion control these foods, because the Eats work on so many different levels for weight loss. If you want to eat an entire package of berries for breakfast, you can! If you wanted to bake sweet potato chips you can eat as many as you want! The possibilities are endless for delicious Eats which are low in calories, keep you feeling full – and are high in the minerals, vitamins, and phytonutrients that your body needs to be healthy, including antioxidants. These foods are unlimited – because the Eats are nature's diet pill.

Eating the Eats, and The Cheats and Eats Lifestyle Programme way of eating as a whole, helps you lose weight across the board by making the process of weight loss natural and easy for your body. By eating three meals a day that contain the protein our body needs to maintain itself, the healthy fats that make us feel satiated, and the Eats that keep us full, reduce our inflammation and stabilise the physiological responses like cortisol and insulin, at every level this programme makes it easy for your body to lose the excess weight.

Unlimited Eats, "Good" Fat, "Traditional" Protein and Cheats on Top!

Every time you look at your plate, it's almost all Eats.

So you now have a sense of what your plate looks like: unlimited Eats, "good" fat, and a "traditional" protein, and of course, your Cheats on top. It's all a part of it.

All that's required for The Cheats and Eats Lifestyle Programme to "work" for you, in terms of diet, is that you focus on your Eats and your Free Cheats (more on this later). This equation combines the work of researchers and doctors who have studied successful weight loss and the experiences of real-life people who have successfully lost weight. It's the marriage of what's been clinically proven to work, and what works in the real world.

On The Cheats and Eats Lifestyle Programme, you don't have to count calories for your Eats, you don't have to worry about fibre or fat, and you don't even have to eliminate foods. We have done the hard work for you. All you have to do is Eat your Eats, which is most of your meal, and limit your Cheats. Seems pretty simple, right?

In Chapter 4, we'll go into the entire plan and show how to start quickly shedding the pounds. The Cheats and Eats Lifestyle Programme has worked for thousands of people, and it will work for you. We've mastered the hardest part of losing weight: making a diet doable in the real world, and making it easy for you to follow through on your intentions and goals to get healthy. As *Men's Health* says, "Abs are made in the kitchen," and 75 per cent of weight loss is making sure you eat your Eats. In the next chapter, we'll show you what makes up the remaining 25 per cent.

CHAPTER 3

Move More –
The Non Negotiable!

Food is the most abused anxiety drug. Exercise is the most underutilised antidepressant.

Maybe you think you can't lose weight because you don't think you have the workout "gene" or because you don't have professional help at the gym. You're not like my best friend from high school who used to work out for three hours every day. You're not like your neighbour, who puts on his running shoes and goes out for a run on Saturday mornings. You think these people aren't like you, are never going to be you, and you'll just get by with whatever you can do.

Or maybe you think you know what to do when you work out. You know that you should lift weights twice a week, do cardio three or four days a week, and do interval training. Maybe you're the type of person who competes in triathlons just for fun, or to see how far you can push yourself.

Whether you're the kind of person who does marathons for fun or the kind of person who thinks you would die trying to run a mile, *fitness fusion*, aka The Cheats and Eats Lifestyle Programme Exercise Plan – will help you not only lose weight, but keep you motivated to move and also help you from being sidelined in the future.

Just like the Diet Fusion concept you learned about in the previous chapter, *Fitness Fusion* combines the best of what's out there into a plan that not only works, but is actually doable in real life.

When you do the right kind of exercise, at the right speed and the right intensity for your individual body, each workout you do will be more productive for weight loss – and once you see those results, the stress you feel about working out will also decrease because you'll know that what you're doing works!

The Four Pillars to Fitness Fusion

You don't have to become a gym rat, or a marathoner, or someone who goes to yoga five times a week in order to make the Cheats and Eats fitness plan work for you. In fact, the opposite is true! We've found that combining the four pillars to fitness fusion is all you need to do in order to make a workout *truly* productive:

- Build your base
- Walk, walk and then do more walking!
- Find the movement and fitness you love
- Confront your stress

1. Building Your Base – Creating YOUR Starting Point

No matter where you are in your health and fitness journey, there will always be a starting point. Knowing that starting point is the first step to improving it. The simple exercise of sitting down and standing up again without holding onto anything is a simple test of muscle strength, endurance and balance. Complete this challenge prior to starting your Fitness Fusion, make a note of your result and re-test every three weeks. You will be surprised at your improvements!

The challenge: 30-second chair test

Sit comfortably on a dining room chair, your feet planted firmly on the ground. Set a stopwatch, and simply stand (without using your hands or arms for support), then sit again (gently) as many times as you can in 30 seconds. A healthy aim for women should be to achieve at least 12 and men 14.

If you find this easy, progress to a softer, lower easy-chair which demands greater strength and balance to get up and down without support, and see how many times you can get up and down out of the chair in 30 seconds.

But where and how do I start?
The reality is we simply need to move more. The official recommendation is to aim to be active daily and to achieve a target of at least two and half hours of physical activity over a week.

Don't put it off until tomorrow or next week. It really doesn't matter where you start, you just need to start! Starting is the hardest, most intimidating part of movement and exercise…but its achievable no matter how small that start is. Do something different TODAY!

Top tips to help you get started:
♦ Don't let intimidation put you off!
It is important to recognise that activity and movement does not mean hitting the gym four times a week! Simply walking for 10 minutes every day will be of benefit to your health, body and mind. Start with walking for 10 continuous minutes. Do this three times a day and eventually aim for 30 continuous minutes daily.

♦ Little and often is key and adherence is the biggest WIN!
Start off small and focus on the words 'regular' rather than 'harder'. Don't expect to go from zero to hero in two days and be realistic with your time management and goal setting. Remember, simply doing 10 minutes of walking every day will drastically improve your health.

♦ Manage your time
Planning time to be active, organising what to eat, getting up earlier in the morning all takes planning and a lot of it! Making activity a priority is a step in the right direction. Small steps = big wins. Don't set yourself up to fail by creating unrealistic goals. Start off small and tick off in your diary when you have completed your task. Charting your progress is incredibly important to see progression.

◆ Find something fun to do

Most of the time it's not what you do, it's how often you do it. If it's not fun, you simply won't want to do it! You have stopped before you have even started! Yes, potentially there are 'more efficient' ways to achieve goals (doing resistance work, compound movements etc.) but if you love 10 pin bowling and you are going to go bowling three times a week…stick to ten pin bowling!

2. Walk, Walk and Then do More Walking!

Walking is hugely underestimated for it's health and fitness benefits. For me, walking is where I clear my head. Something about the methodical steps and my heart beat makes it incredibly relaxing.

Why is walking great?
◆ Walking is free
◆ Walking requires ZERO equipment
◆ Walking can be done at any time of day
◆ Walking can be done anywhere in the world
◆ You don't need to be fit to walk
◆ Walking can be done alone or with a friend or in a group

What are the benefits of walking?
◆ Walking helps to improves your mood
Being active and walking helps boosts the levels of potent brain chemicals like serotonin, dopamine, and norepinephrine – which make you feel happy!

◆ Walking promotes healthy muscles
Simply put; use it or lose it! The less we use our muscles and joints the shorter our muscles will get and the tighter our bodies will be. Walking is a great weight-bearing exercise and assists our muscle flexibility and strength, in turn allowing us to perform daily activities with more ease.

10,000 Steps a Day
To be moderately active, the average adult should complete two and half hours of activity each week. This sounds a lot! In actual fact it is

half an hour of exercise every single day. The 10,000 daily step target equates to the same amount of moderate activity.

To start with 10,000 can sound a lot. But it's important at the beginning to take note of your current step level and try to slowly increase it. If you are currently walking 4,000 steps a day, to get to 10,000 may be too larger target. Increase by 2,000 steps at a time. When you are comfortably reaching a daily target of 6,000 it is then time to increase it to 8,000 and so on.

If you are already walking 10,000 steps a day it is important to set a higher target to challenge yourself. Aim for 12,000 and then increase by 2,000 and so on. Simply including a 30 minute walk into your daily routine will help you on your way to 10,000 steps. This can be broken down into smaller chunks initially. Such as three, 10-minute walks, but eventually, try to walk for 30 continuous minutes.

It is also important to remember that getting your step level up doesn't mean only going for long walks in the park! Try and use your feet as often as you can. It really does make a difference!

- Opt to walk up the stairs rather than taking the lift or escalator.
- Wash your own car rather than taking it to garage and watching someone else do it.
- Sweep the leaves up in your garden, rather than employing a gardener to do it.
- Walk to get a morning coffee from a coffee shop 10 minutes away rather than at the end of your street.

3. Finding the Movement and Fitness You Love

If you really embrace the ideas from the first two fitness pillars, this third step will probably come easily. You will find that you *want to move more*, and you will be open to the possibility that exercise doesn't have to be boring, that it can be fun.

When you enjoy the feeling of exercise, you are motivated for life. When you start doing a workout that you like, you may begin to realise why some people claim to love exercise. And that's because those people know about flow.

Flow: How to Make Exercise Fun

Although athletes call flow different things – being in the zone and runner's high – flow is when your body and mind come together to make exercise engaging, fulfilling and entertaining. Being in a flow state is an easy way to become even more physically fit than you ever thought possible, because it makes exercise doable both physically and mentally. While you'll notice that flow states require you to slow down at first, the more flow workouts you do the faster you will get without injury and without wanting to quit.

It's easiest to experience flow when you are doing an activity that you love. If you aren't enjoying your workout routine now, think of what you liked doing when you were younger. For example, when I was growing up I danced almost every day: tap, jazz, ballet, but at some point, I just gave it up. So I bought the video game Dance Party. I can do it by myself, or suggest it when people come over. I bought Wii Tennis for the same reason. I don't need a court, or a partner, or good weather, just the Wii. And when I'm doing those things, I'm moving, which is what really matters.

Jonathan Fields, who specialises in and has written books about flow, says that being in flow requires absorption and mental focus – while still having fun. Most mainstream fitness routines prevent flow by being activities that are really boring – a treadmill is a great example. The reason treadmills have televisions that most people plug into and tune out on is because the exercise is so boring!

In contrast, running outside, or better yet, running on a trail, requires your full attention and engages you. You have to concentrate on where you're running, or else you'll run into a tree or stumble on a rock and fall. Because you're outside, your surroundings change, keeping you interested in what's happening around you. That mental engagement is rewarding and satisfying – which encourages you to keep going, to finish the workout, and especially to come back for more another day.

By its very nature, flow is a bit mystifying until it happens to you. But there are eight requirements to flow, which Jonathan Fields, the founder of the Good Life Project, first explained to me (which I've included below). These eight stages have to happen in combination with each other (nearly simultaneously) in order for you to enter a flow state. It's important to note, though, that flow isn't just for exercise: it can happen at work, when you're in conversation with a good friend, when you're playing a musical instrument, or knitting a scarf, or practising a craft, or writing a story, or doing anything that requires both creativity and focus.

The Eight Stages of Flow

1. Clear Goals
You know what you want to achieve and what the rules of the activity are, even if you set those boundaries for yourself. For example, a tennis player knows the rules of the game and wants to beat their opponent; if you're walking, you could have set a goal of being able to walk faster than before, or simply to walk for a certain length of time.

2. High Concentration
You're focused solely on what you're doing, not what else you have to do during the day or what has been weighing on your mind prior to the activity. You're intensely focused on what you're doing and how it is making your body feel.

3. It's Hard But Not Tough
There's a balance between the activity requiring the skills you already have and being challenging at the same time. So, if you are playing tennis you could have a worthy opponent who is slightly better than you; if you're walking, you're keeping a slightly faster pace than normal, but can still breathe.

4. You're In Control
You feel secure and relaxed psychologically while doing the activity. You're not worried about what you look like, what obstacles may be in your path, or what the other people around you think about you or what you're doing.

5. It Feels Effortless
Though the activity may look strenuous to someone else, it doesn't cause any strain to you. And honestly, you realise that you don't need to think about what you're doing all that much while doing it.

6. No Perception of Time

You feel like you could go on forever, or that the amount of time you've spent exercising feels like half of what is showing on your watch or smartphone.

7. A Feeling of Unity

There is no mental room for worry, fear, distraction or rumination. You feel at peace with your performance, or if participating with others in a group activity, how your team is performing as a whole. You feel deeply connected to what you're doing, like your performance and yourself are one and the same.

8. Immediately Gratifying

When you're finished with the activity, you feel like you could go out and do it again – or want to, just because you want to replicate the feeling you had while you were doing the exercise. This can also happen while you are doing the activity – creating the feeling that you never want to stop.

Each stage of flow can happen independently of the others, so if you decide to try a new exercise, try to be conscious of how you are feeling. If you lose perception of time, or find yourself feeling super pumped up and wanting to do that activity again when you finish your workout, those are great indicators that whatever activity you're doing could induce a flow state should you keep doing it.

While it doesn't matter what kind of exercise or activity you are doing when you are able to get into flow, being in a flow state helps your body supercharge its fat burning (and lower cortisol) because you're moving at the right pace and you are totally relaxed. If you've never been in flow state before, start with a mental or physical activity that is appealing and easy for you to do. It can be drawing. It can be tennis. Something that makes you feel great.

Walking can often induce flow states and provide you with the mental space you need to clear the mental clutter that's been causing stress. As a general rule, classes are more inclined to create flow states than your usual gym equipment workout. Any activity you think that you "should" do, but worry that you might get hurt doing, or really dislike, is an activity that is the opposite of flow. You are in flow when you feel great and you're doing well.

Zumba, yoga, team sports, and even cardio body-sculpting classes can induce group flow states – where everyone in the room is in flow – which have even more powerful effects on weight loss.

4. Confronting Your Stress

Stress holds you back from losing weight just as much, if not more, than sitting on your couch would. The moment you feel stressed, your body responds by releasing cortisol.

Five Miles or Five Minutes

Let's say you were super-motivated one morning and went out for a five-mile run. Your hormones would change as you exercised – especially cortisol – but you would also experience the positive effects of a physical workout like better cardiovascular fitness, improved insulin sensitivity, increasing your lean body mass (muscle) and of course decreasing fat (as long as you're fat burning).

Now let's pretend that instead of going for a run, you looked at Facebook, saw that your ex is getting married, and proceeded to totally stress out about it for five minutes. Your body would react to this stress in the same way it would have reacted to the exercise, but experience none of the physical benefits of the five-mile run. Instead, it would only receive the negative effects of your hormones at work, including increased belly fat.

Your brain and your body simply can't tell the difference between physiological stress caused by physical activity (the five-mile run) and mental stress (the ex getting married). Your body reacts to both situations, physiologically, the same way: it increases cortisol, which starts breaking down your muscle in order to make new glucose (sugar), and it signals to the body that it needs to preserve all of its blood sugar for the brain.

Unlike during exercise where your blood sugar might actually be low because of an actual demand for energy, when you are psychologically stressed, your body doesn't need all that extra blood sugar and so stores it as fat, usually into your belly (cortisol's favourite place to deposit fat cells). Think of extreme physiological stress as adding petrol to the tank of your car but never starting it!

Stress within our body, whether it's physical or mental, is the worst workout you can do when trying to lose weight. I see more people putting undue stress on themselves by giving away their power than anything else.

We can give away our power by putting ourselves down in front of others ("I can't eat that cake today – you should have seen what a fatty I was last night!"), by saying yes to something when we want to say no or otherwise trying to please people at our own expense. Either way, we decrease the amount of personal power we have to make positive changes for ourselves in our lives.

When you don't stand up for yourself, your dreams and goals, or what you really want and deserve, you give away your power and essentially take a step back from achieving what you really want and becoming who you really want to be. And, from a weight-loss perspective, all that brooding will hold you back from what your body needs, physiologically, to shed fat.

So, a great piece of advice that I want you to keep in mind while you're on The Cheats and Eats Lifestyle Programme is from personal development coach Joshua Wayne: **"What other people think of me is none of my business." It's the truth! You can't control what people think of you, so why bother wondering about it? It only holds you back.**

The more you concentrate on what you *can* control – and the less mind space you give things that you can't – the more you will feel like you can succeed on this plan. You can't help that the magical yoga class is not at the right time for you. But you can control what you put in your mouth and how much you move throughout the day.

I am no stranger to massive stress. As an entrepreneur, and as a wife, mother and daughter, there are a million stresses I encounter each and every day. But I've learned that how your body handles stress is directly related to how you react to it, and the way you're reacting to it now is probably keeping that weight on. At some point you have to make a choice and stop dwelling on the things you can't control.

At some point you have to acknowledge the damage stress is doing to your body and your goals. You have to say to yourself, "I'm either going to keep stressing out and keep this weight on" or "I'm going to react differently" and learn how to change the way you react.

Tips and Tricks

It's really hard to stop stressing out but you have to do it to lose the weight. It's not a "nice to have", it's a *must* and it's a critical component of The Cheats and Eats Lifestyle Programme. What works for me? My first trick: "What other people think of me is none of my business." That works when I think someone may be critical of something I'm doing, or when someone actually says something critical to my face.

The second trick I use when I start to freak out is that I ask myself, "Is there anything I can control here?" Most of the time there isn't, and once you realise that, it instantly diffuses the situation.

The third trick is a relaxation exercise I learned from sleep experts Mitchell and Olga Stevko. Sit down, take a deep breath, and focus on a colour that relaxes you. Put whatever stresses you out in the middle of that colour, whether it's a friend or a family member or a task or whatever. Give it an image in your mind and then make it smaller and smaller. You can even "shoot" it with a gun or a cannon if you like. As the stressor disappears, replace it with an image or an idea that makes you happy – and make that image bigger and bigger. This might sound woo-woo but I find that it's the easiest way to stop stress in its tracks.

What all three of these tricks do is allow for you to control your reaction over an external force, person or situation that you can't control. That switches the channel for your brain – there's nothing for it to fix. You can also treat things that stress you out, or experiences that are negative, the same way you treat television shows you don't like: turn it off, change the channel. You can literally change the channel in your mind by thinking of something else.

When I start thinking about things I can't control, I joke to my husband and my friends that the monkeys in my brain are swinging around wildly. I say, "Uh-oh, the monkeys are gathering for the big bash." It allows me to see that the thoughts are out of control – and picturing them as crazy monkeys helps diminish the power of what I was ruminating over.

These are just a few solutions, but I promise that the more open you are to new suggestions that can help you solve problems, overcome obstacles to weight loss, and relieve stress, the more likely your pounds will drop off. It's like everything else in the book: if your solutions were working for you, you wouldn't be reading this book. So, don't be afraid to try one of these exercises, or any other stress-reduction techniques you read about in magazines or whatever. Find what works for you, and use it – no matter how ridiculous it may seem to other people. Because the better you are able to manage your stress, the better you'll be able to keep the pounds off.

Change Your Mind, Change Your Weight

When you stop beating yourself up, you take yourself off the mental treadmill – and you decrease your stress and hormones stress triggers. Not worrying incessantly when you skip a workout about whether you'll gain weight, or about what your ex-boyfriend is doing or someone is saying about you, all helps your body maintain the weight.

It's totally fine to miss a workout every once in a while. It's not the end of the world and you're certainly not a failure. Your weight loss goals will not be diminished by not going for a walk one day or by skipping a Zumba class that doesn't fit into your schedule. When you decide to de-stress your life and don't worry about how you're not working out as much as you once did, you will lose more weight.

Our tendency is to be self-deprecating for all the things we can't do or aren't able to do. This plan trys to shift that focus and take you away from negativity toward yourself and more toward positivity. When you think about exercise, concentrate on your base: What can you do? What do you like to do? And when can you do it?

By focusing on that, instead of churning and burning on some machine for an arbitrary amount of time an arbitrary number of days each week, you'll be able to not only enjoy the exercise you're doing but you'll also see the results on your body. It's much more powerful to concentrate on how great you are. Sure, you should understand the negative – about yourself, about exercise, about life – but embracing all the awesome things about you and understanding that there's a balance is the key to chilling out and allowing The Cheats and Eats Lifestyle Programme programme, as a whole, to work for you.

And one final note: being stressed out and ruminating makes it really hard to lose weight, because it could be the biggest reason you might not be sleeping.

A Magic Pill: Sleep

Sleep may be the most important single thing you can do to easily lose weight. Some experts even believe that getting enough sleep nightly is even more important than diet and exercise for health and longevity. A study has shown that people eat 35 per cent more when sleep deprived than when they are fully rested. A lack of sleep could be a significant reason why you feel "hungry all day" – because your cortisol is raised when you don't get enough rest.

The most important step you can take right now to establish healthy sleep patterns is to know what your "sleep number" is. How many hours per night do you need to be rested and energised during the day? According to the Stanford Sleep Centre, it's between seven and nine hours a night. Your number is probably the amount of sleep you are sleeping each night by the end of a week's holiday. Once you know your sleep number, try this: set your alarm for the same time every day, *including weekends*, that gives you that amount of time to sleep. So, for instance, if you need eight hours of sleep and you have to get up by 7 a.m. for work, you should be in bed at 11 p.m. and set your alarm for 7 a.m. Remember, if you're not sleeping, you're snacking all day.

The most common issue that people face with sleep is the inability to stop racing thoughts while lying in bed, and calming the mind. I call this "calming my monkeys". I know everything is Ok when I have a visual of the monkeys no longer partying. They're sitting and watching TV. That relaxation exercise is one of the greatest tools I have. If I'm still awake after that, I try not to get mad because I know the monkeys have to do a workout before I'll be able to sleep.

Also, a side note, please don't eat within at least two to three hours before going to bed. Set your alarm for going to bed, just like you set your alarm to wake up. Don't go to bed with the TV. Read instead.

The Truth About Muscles

A lot of people (especially women) focus on cardiovascular workouts and weight-bearing strength training (Pilates, yoga, etc.) instead of traditional weight-lifting workouts. But the truth is that combining strength training with cardiovascular workouts will not only encourage your body to lose weight, it also makes you look better in clothes and increases your overall fitness.

Doing a resistance based workout two to three times a week helps your body grow its lean muscle mass, which is good because lean muscle mass is "expensive" for your body to maintain. Having it consumes a lot of energy.

When your body has more lean muscle mass, it has a faster metabolism and burns more calories (even at rest) than if it had less because it's sucking more petrol from your engine, and doing it quicker. Not to mention that lean muscle mass makes you look thin without looking skinny. In fact, most of the people you think are "naturally thin" probably look that way because they have healthy amounts of lean muscle mass.

You can develop lean muscle mass by lifting weights. Strength-training is actually one of the best fat-burning workouts available, because it increases metabolism so much after you're done working out. And, last but not least, if you're worried that lifting weights will make you look like a bodybuilder, I can tell you from experience that it won't happen.

The Three-Week Workout Plan

Disclaimer: Please Use Common Sense

Listen to your body. Starting a new exercise routine will place different demands on your body. If you have any concerns, check with your GP first and stop if you experience any pain or discomfort.

Follow The Cheats and Eats Lifestyle Programme Fitness Plan for the next three weeks. Six out of seven days are structured movement days. To achieve the best results, aim to complete the full programme three times a week, making sure you have an active rest day in-between.

Each week the programme will increase slightly in intensity. If you are not quite ready for this increase, simply repeat the week you are on as many times as you need before moving to the next level. At the end of the three weeks we have created a Cheats and Eats System Maintenance Fitness Plan. This final plan is of a similar structure to the previous three weeks, but includes a few additional exercises.

Day 1	Day 2	Day 3	Day 4	Day 5	Day 6	Day 7
Cheats and Eats System Fitness Plan	Active Rest	Cheats and Eats System Fitness Plan	Active Rest	Cheats and Eats System Fitness Plan	Social Cardio – Finding your Flow	Day Off

Active rest or recovery simply means 'lower level' movement. Great examples of active rest are walking, swimming, stretching, yoga and pilates.

One day a week is allocated to 'social cardio', the perfect opportunity to 'find your flow' (see pages 58–61) . This should be sweaty and fun and possibly with a friend or in a group. Great examples are cycling, a game of tennis or going to a Zumba class.

To Start – The Warm Up

Try to think of exercise as a front, middle and end. These are the warm up, the workout and the cool down.

Warming up is incredibly important and is often overlooked. The warm up prepares the brain and body for what is to come during the workout. Slowly increasing the heart rate, and in turn your blood flow, will help mobilise the joints and lengthen the muscles. A good warm up also reduces the chance of injury. We cannot expect the body to go from 0–60 instantly – think of it as a car that needs warming up on an icy day!

The Cool Down

Another important element of your workout. It is essential following your workout to decrease intensity levels to bring down your heart rate and ultimately bring your body back to a restful state. Cooling down and completing some dynamic stretches will aid recovery by returning the muscles to their normal length, will help any muscles soreness, will help reduce levels of lactic acid in the blood and will generally help your body along with it's repairing and recovery process.

WEEK ONE

Warm Up
Complete 10 repetitions of the below seven moves in order. Repeat three times. Try to exaggerate each move by making them as 'big' as possible.

1. Knee Hugs
• Stand tall with feet hip width apart
• Raise one foot off the floor and hug the knee into to your chest
• Slowly lower leg back to the ground
• Alternate

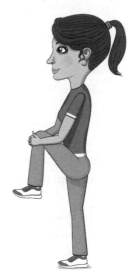

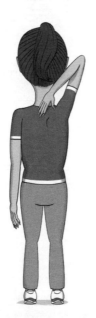

2. Tricep Taps
• Stand tall with feet hip width apart
• Lift arm in front of you, take it high in the air above your head
• Try to keep your elbow high, bend at the elbow and tap your palm between shoulder blades
• Return to start position and alternate
• Try to keep head looking forward

3. Toe Touches

- Stand tall with feet hip width apart
- Move one leg out in front of you
- Bend at the hips and reach forward with hand to touch the toe on the same side*
- Return to standing and alternate

*Don't worry if you cannot touch your toes!

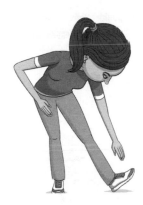

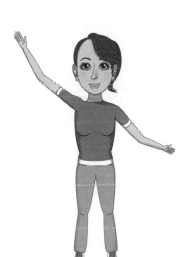

4. Chest Opens

- Stand tall with feet hip width apart
- Lift arms out in front of you at shoulder height, palms touching
- Open arms out wide to stretch the chest, then return to centre to clap hands in front of the body
- Repeat

5. Heel to Bum

- Stand tall with feet hip width apart
- Bending your knee, flick your heel up behind you as if you are trying to touch your bum
- Return to standing. Repeat alternating the leg

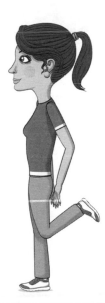

6. Shoulder Rolls

- Stand tall with feet hip width apart
- Place hands on shoulders (left hand, left shoulder
  – right hand, right shoulder)
- Draw circles with your elbows

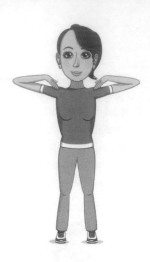

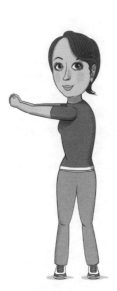

7. Torso Twists

- Stand tall with feet hip width apart, knee's
  slightly bent
- Keep your head looking forward for the entire
  movement
- Lift your arms to chest height and clasp hands
  together
- Slowly rotate the torso and your arms from left to
  right whilst maintaining eyes looking forward

The Workout

Complete 15 of each exercise below in order. Take a short rest at the end of the exercises and try
and repeat a further 1–2 times.

1. Half Squat to Chair

- Stand tall, feet hip width apart, about a foot
  and a half in front of a sturdy chair
- Gently lower your bottom onto the chair
- Push through the heels to stand back up and
  squeeze your butt cheeks at the top

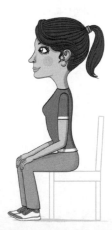

2. Towel Raise

- Stand tall, one foot in front of the other
- Take a hand towel in both hands, pulling it tight
- Start with the towel touching the thighs. Slowly lift your arms out in front of you, keeping arms stretched and keeping tension on the towel at all times
- Lift all the way up, high above your head
- Slowly lower back to the start position, keeping torso braced and towel taut
- Repeat

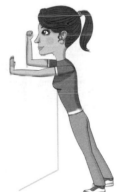

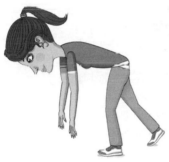

3. Backward Steps

- Stand tall with feet hip width apart
- Take one foot behind you and step backwards. At the same time, tilt forwards from the hips, bend your legs to try and touch the floor in front of you
- Keep your body weight in your front foot
- Drive through the heel of the front foot, and return upright to standing
- Alternate leg
- This move should look like you are simply picking something up from the floor

4. Plank Press Against Wall

- Stand tall around two feet away from a wall
- Take your hands to the wall, hands directly under your shoulders
- Bracing your abdominals lower your right side so the right elbow is on the wall, then lower the left side. At this point both elbows are on the wall
- Keeping tummy tight and with as little movement through the hips, place your right hand where your right elbow was, then do the same with the left, to return to starting position
- Complete all reps on right side, then switch to do the left

The Cool Down

Complete 10 slow repetitions of each of the warm up moves in order. Repeat two times. Work slowly through the moves and exaggerate each move by making them as 'big' as possible.

Knee Hugs – Tricep Taps – Toe Touches – Chest Opens – Heel to Bum – Shoulder Rolls – Torso Twists

WEEK TWO

Complete your warm up as before: Knee Hugs - Tricep Taps - Toe Touches - Chest Opens - Heel to Bum - Shoulder Rolls - Torso Twists

The Workout
Complete 15 of each exercise below in order. Take a short rest at the end of the exercises and try and repeat a further 1–2 times.

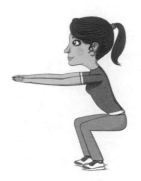

1. Half Body Weight Squat
- Stand tall with feet hip width apart
- Sit back as if sitting on an imaginary chair, pushing arms out in front
- Keep your body weight in your heels (you should be able to lift your big toe in your shoe)
- Push through your heels to return to standing
- Try to keep the weight in your heels and keep your chest up as much as you can (try not to look down)

2. Plank Press On Step from Knees
- On the floor with knees bent, using a box/step/low chair in front of you
- Place hands on the step, hands directly under shoulders
- Your trunk should be solid and your body weight should be in the hands
- Lower right side so right elbow is on the step, then lower left side. At this point both elbows should be on the step
- With tummy tight and with as little movement as possible through the hips, place right hand where right elbow was, then do the same with the left, to return to start position
- Complete all reps on right side, then switch to do the left side

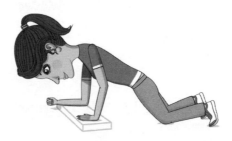

3. Knee Up and Knee Down

- Stand tall with feet hip width apart
- Step one foot backwards and your lower knee to the floor
- Bring the other knee down to join it on the floor (both knees are now on the floor)
- Raise one foot back in front, push through your heel and return to standing

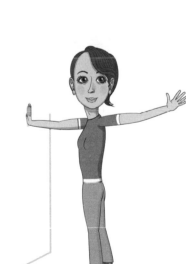

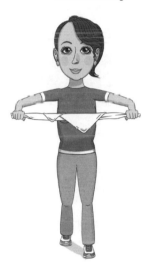

4. Towel High Row

- Take a hand towel in both hands
- Stand tall, one foot in front of the other
- Stretch arms out in front of you at chest height, with tension on the towel (imagine you are trying to snap the towel in half)
- Keeping the towel at chest height and elbows high, slowly drag the towel back to touch your chest (keeping tension on the towel at all times)
- Slowly return to the start position, keeping torso braced and towel taut
- Repeat

5. Plank Rotations on Wall

- Stand tall, an arm's distance away from a wall
- Take hands to the wall, directly under the shoulders
- Bracing the abdominals, lift right hand off the wall, out to the side, and then behind you all at shoulder height. Opening your body to the side
- Let your eyes follow your right hand
- Slowly and under control, lower right hand back to the wall
- Alternate with the left side

Complete the **Cool Down** as before – Knee Hugs – Tricep Taps – Toe Touches – Chest Opens – Heel to Bum – Shoulder Rolls – Torso Twists

WEEK THREE

Complete the **Warm Up** as per week one – Knee Hugs – Tricep Taps – Toe Touches – Chest Opens – Heel to Bum – Shoulder Rolls – Torso Twists

The Workout

Complete 15 of each exercise below in order. Take a short rest at the end of the exercises and try and repeat a further 1–2 times.

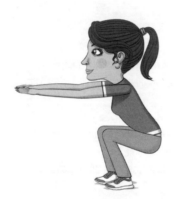

1. Full Squat
• Stand tall with feet hip width apart
• Sit back as if sitting on a low imaginary chair, pushing your arms out in front
• Keep your body weight in your heels (you should be able to lift you big toe in your shoe)
• Push through your heels to return to standing, squeezing your butt cheeks at the top
• The aim here is for full depth squat keeping weight in heels, chest lifted whilst getting as low as you can in the squat

2. Plank Press on Step from Knees
• On the floor with knees bent, using a bench/step in front of you
• Place hands on the bench, hands directly under shoulders
• Your trunk should be solid and your body weight should be in the hands
• Lower right side so right elbow is on the bench, then lower left side. At this point both elbows should be on the bench

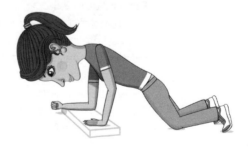

• With tummy tight and with as little movement as possible through the hips, place right hand where right elbow was, then do the same with the left, to return to start position
• Complete all reps on right side, then switch to do the left side

3. Knee Up/Knee Down with Twist

- Stand tall with feet hip width apart
- Step right foot backwards and lower knee to touch the floor
- At the same time, rotate your right hand to touch your left knee, your left arm should move backwards behind you
- Drive through left foot to return to standing, bring arms back to your sides
- Alternate, take left leg backwards, rotate torso so left hand touches right knee, your right arm should move behind you
- Keep torso lifted

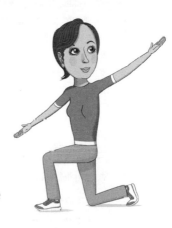

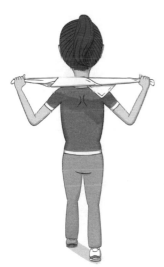

4. Towel Raise and Lat Pull

- Take a hand towel in both hands
- Stand tall, one foot in front of the other
- Start with the towel touching the thighs, slowly lift out in front of you (keeping tension on the towel at all times) until your arms are stretched out high in the air above your head
- Slowly lower the towel behind your head
- Slowly bring the towel back above your head, then drag the towel back to the thighs
- Keep torso braced and tension on the towel throughout. Repeat

5. Plank Rotations on Knees and Step

- On the floor with a box/step/low chair in front of you
- On your knees, place hands on the bench in front of you, hands directly under shoulders
- Your trunk should be solid and your body weight should be in the hands
- Lift right hand off the bench, out to the side, and then behind you all at shoulder height. Opening your body to the side. Let your eyes follow your right hand
- Slowly and under control, lower right hand back to the bench
- Repeat with the left side

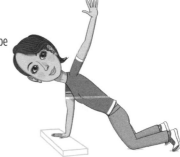

6. Mountain Climber Hands on Wall

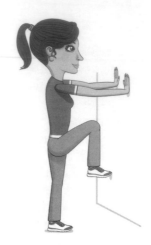

- Stand tall, an arm's length away from the wall
- Take hands to the wall, hands directly under shoulders
- Bracing the abdominals, drag one knee towards your chest
- Slowly return the foot to the floor and alternate

Complete the **Cool Down** as before – Knee Hugs – Tricep Taps – Toe Touches – Chest Opens – Heel to Bum – Shoulder Rolls – Torso Twists

WEEK FOUR

On-Going Maintenance Programme

Complete the **Warm Up** as per week one – Knee Hugs – Tricep Taps – Toe Touches – Chest Opens – Heel to Bum – Shoulder Rolls – Torso Twists

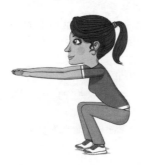

The Workout

1. Full squat

- Stand tall with feet hip width apart
- Sit back as if sitting on a low imaginary chair
- Keep body weight in your heels and hands/arms lifted (you should be able to lift you big toe in your shoe)
- Push through your heels to return to standing

2. Plank Press on Floor, on Knees

- Start on the floor with knees bent
- Place hands on the floor in front of you, hands directly under shoulders. Your trunk should be solid and your weight should be in the hands
- Lower right side so right elbow is on the floor, then lower left side. At this point both elbows should be on the floor

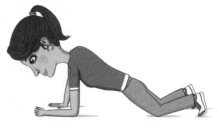

- With tummy tight and with as little movement as possible through the hips, place right hand where right elbow was, then do the same with the left, to return to the start position. Complete all repetitions on right side, then switch to do the left

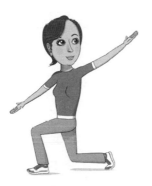

3. Full Backward Stepping Lunge with Twist (Thumbs Turned Out)

- Stand tall with feet hip width apart, arms directly out to your sides at shoulder height, palms up, thumbs pointing backwards
- Take a big step backwards with the right foot, bend the back knee and dip it towards the floor
- At the same time, rotate your right hand to touch your left knee, your left arm should move backwards behind you
- Drive through the outer foot to return to standing, bring your arms back to your sides
- Alternate, so side lunge left leg backwards, rotate torso so left hand touches right knee, left arm should move behind you. Keep torso lifted throughout

4. Towel High Row, Raise and Lat Pull

- Hold a towel in both hands, stand tall, one foot in front of the other
- Start with the towel touching the thighs, slowly lift out in front of you to chest height (keeping it taut)
- With the towel at chest height and elbows high, slowly drag the towel back to touch your chest
- Slowly return to the start position
- Repeat lifting towel in front of you high above your head then slowly lower the towel behind your head
- Slowly bring the towel high above your head, then drag the towel back to the thighs. Repeat
- Keep torso braced and the towel taut throughout

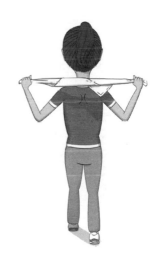

5. Plank rotations on knees

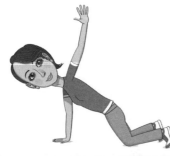

- On the floor with knees bent
- Place hands on the floor in front of you, hands directly under shoulders. Your trunk should be solid and your body weight should be in the hands
- Lift right hand off the floor, out to the side, and then behind you all at shoulder height. Opening your body to the side
- Let your eyes follow your right hand
- Slowly and under control, lower right hand back to the floor
- Alternate now with the left side

6. Mountain Climber, Hands on Floor

• Start on the floor in a high plank position with your hands directly under shoulders
• Your trunk should be solid and your body weight should be in the hands
• Bracing the abdominals, drag one knee towards your chest
• Slowly return the foot to the floor and alternate

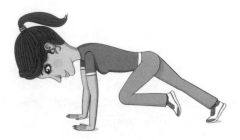

7. Simple Four-Point Superman

• Start on the floor with knees bent, directly under your hips
• Place hands on the floor in front of you, hands directly under shoulders
• Keeping your abdominals braced, slowly push your right leg behind you at the same time lifting your left arm out in front
• Slowly and under control, lower both back to the start position then alternate
• Focus on stretching the arms and legs rather than lifting up. Ensure your lower back doesn't arch and your abdominals remain braced

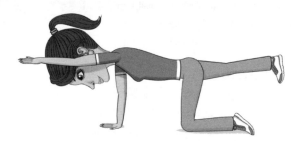

Complete the **Cool Down** as per week one – Knee Hugs – Tricep Taps – Toe Touches – Chest Opens – Heel to Bum – Shoulder Rolls – Torso Twists

What are you waiting for?

If just reading about the exercise plan tires you out make sure you start off small. Remember any movement you do today is more than you did yesterday!

PART TWO

Lose Weight, Fast

The Cheats and Eats Lifestyle Programme Explained

Eats: You Can Never Be Too Rich, Too Thin, or Eat Too Many Eats

Cheats: Keep All the Foods You Love to Eat, Just Limit the Cheats

Finish each day and be done with it. You have done what you could. Some blunders and absurdities no doubt crept in; forget them as soon as you can. Tomorrow is a new day...

– RALPH WALDO

What has become clear from listening to people who have followed The Cheats and Eats Lifestyle Programme is that when people start slow, change becomes doable and great things happen. That's why we've created The Cheats and Eats Lifestyle Programme so you can work at your own pace, incorporating the Eats and limiting your Cheats, to get to your goals instead of feeling like you're destined to fail on some regimented, restrictive, all-or-nothing plan.

 I follow The Cheats and Eats Lifestyle Programme about 80 per cent of the time, and keep trying to move closer to the ideal. I feel great when I follow the programme closely. I have been doing this for about six months and have lost about fifteen pounds.   – Gail

The Cheat Sheet is the key to The Cheats and Eats Lifestyle Programme, and it is very simple. The Cheat Sheet is a **list** – Eats are on the left side and Cheats on the right.

Your number one rule, that you absolutely must follow, is this: You *eat* the Eats. As much as you want. The eats are the absolute answer, the magic bullet – because when you eat the Eats you gain control over everything else you eat. I really mean that. The Eats keep you full so that when you do eat Cheats – because we all will – you're not going to overdo it or be at the mercy of a ridiculously huge craving.

You've gotta eat the Eats to get rid of those pounds…and the more Eats you eat, the more weight you'll lose. So, eat, eat, eat, eat, eat, *eat, eat, eat.* **Eat your Eats!**

Now to the part you've all been waiting for: the Cheats. What is a Cheat? A Cheat is food that is listed on the right side of the list, something that isn't going to help you lose weight but that you want, that you really enjoy, or that you crave. On The Cheats and Eats

Much easier to follow than other diets/trackers/changes I've tried, especially not having to keep track of every single morsel of food I eat.

"Only keeping track of Cheats is *so* much easier, and I always know I can eat off the free list if I'm hungry without feeling guilty!

"I knew there had to be something more out there than simply counting every single calorie and depriving myself constantly . . . I just couldn't find anything that accomplished that *and* actually fit into my life.

– A. J. K

Lifestyle Programme, you absolutely are *not* denied. You can eat any food you want, at any time, any place. We've done the work for you so you can eat whatever you want and still lose weight. Eating some Cheats on a regular basis will keep you from developing massive cravings because no foods are off limits. You only count the calories in each Cheat, and limit the number of Cheats you have overall throughout the day. Cheating and eating takes nothing off your table.

The Cheats and Eats Lifestyle Programme is simple. There's no need to count how much fat, fibre or sugar is in any food you eat. Eat the Eats and limit your Cheats, plain and simple. Let's begin with the Eats. You get to eat as many Eats as you want, at any time. The Eats are unlimited. Don't worry about having a second, third, or fourth serving of any Eats on the list.

You get to eat any food you want in the form of Cheats as well. What exactly is a *Cheat*? A Cheat is the equivalent of 100 calories. It could be 100 calories of cheese, 100 calories of bacon, 100 calories of pizza, 100 calorie snack pack, 100 calories of whatever. While 50 calories = ½ a cheat (or 0.5). You don't need to worry about anything other than the number of calories in what you eat of Cheats. We don't measure it any other way. There are no other special exceptions you have to remember. Only that one Cheat = 100 calories.

In the beginning, you get 10 Cheats a day. We'll outline a full three-week plan for you and though we'll get into the week-by-week details soon, for now just keep having 10 Cheats per day in your mind. Some of you will find it hard to stick to 10 Cheats a day, and others will find it easy to eat 10 or perhaps even fewer Cheats. I find that when I am "on track" I eat about six Cheats per day. You might be thinking, that's only 600 calories! But keep in mind that I'm eating a significant higher number than that because I'm eating mostly from the Eats side. I know that no one could be full only eating Cheats; I'm focused on my unlimited Eats. The main focus I want you to have is to maximize your Eats (the left column of the Cheat Sheet) and to keep track of your Cheats (on the right). Eventually, we'll minimise the frequency of Cheats, but you don't have to worry about that right now. Just focus on eating!

I told you it was simple, right? Well, over the next few pages is what the Cheat Sheet looks like. Think of this as your menu. You get to eat whatever you want of the Eats, on the left side, in whatever quantities you want. *And* you get to choose 10 Cheats of 100 calories each from the right side.

THE CHEAT SHEET

Vegetables!

An asterisk denotes best bang for your buck: these are
full of nutrition, and will keep you feeling full, too!

*Artichokes
*Asparagus
Aubergine
Bamboo Shoots
Beetroot
*Broccoli
*Brussel sprouts
*Cabbage, all
  varieties
Celeriac
Carrots
Cassava
*Cauliflower
*Celery
Chilli peppers
Courgettes
*Cucumber
*Endive
Fennel
*Garlic
*Green beans

*Green peppers
Jerusalem artichoke
*Kale
Kohlrabi
*Leeks
*Lettuce
*Mixed greens
*Mushrooms
*Mustard greens
*Okra
Onions, all kinds
  including
  Bermuda, red
  onions, yellow
  onions, white,
  sweet
Parsnips
*Peas
Pumpkin
*Radicchio
Radishes

*Rocket
Salsify
*Seaweed, all varieties
Shallots
*Mangetout
*Spinach
*Sprouts, all varieties
Spring greens
*Spring onions
*Sugar snap peas
Squash, all kinds
Sweet peppers
Sweet potatoes
Taro
Tomatoes, all colours
Turnips
*Watercress
Yams

Drinks

Black tea (after first cup it's a
  cheat)
Coffee (after first cup it's a cheat)
Green tea

Herbal tea
Oolong tea
Water
White tea

Wheat and Yeast Products

Breads, bagels, etc.
Cakes
Chocolate
Cookies
Crackers
Crisps
Fried foods
Gluten-free products, all kinds

Most snacks (including pretzels, low-fat bars, granola and popcorn)
Oven chips
Pasta, all kinds
Pizza
Sweets

Dairy Products

Butter
Buttermilk
Cheese, all kinds (including cream cheese)
Cream
Crème fraîche
Eggnog

Ice cream
Milk
Sour cream
Soymilk
Whipped cream
Yogurt

Drinks

Alcohol
All no-calorie drinks, including diet sodas. (If you want to eat chemicals, you'll have to Cheat to do it.)
Any drink that has added flavours or preservatives

Beer
Black coffee and tea after your first cup
Soft drinks, all
Spirits, all kinds
Wine

THE CHEAT SHEET

Best Fruits!
Always unlimited and organic is best

Blackberries	Gooseberries	Pomegranates
Blueberries	Grapefruit	Raspberries
Cranberries	Lemon	Rhubarb
Currants	Lime	Strawberries

More Fruit!
Each day your first serving from the below list is an Eat and after that serving, these fruits become a Cheat

Apples	Mangos	Plums
Apricots	Mangosteens	Prunes
Bananas	Melons	Pomelo
Cherries	Nectarines	Quinces
Custard apples	Olives	Raisins
Dates	Oranges	Rambutans
Figs	Papayas	Sapodilla
Grapes	Peaches	Starfruit
Gooseberries	Pears	Tamarinds
Guava	Persimmons	Tangerines
Kiwi fruit	Pineapple	
Kumquats	Plantains	

Eat Your Beans!
(If using tinned beans, make sure you rinse the beans, otherwise there is a lot of sodium)

Adzuki beans	Cannellini beans	Lentils
Black beans	Chickpeas	Mung beans
Black-eyed peas	Gungo peas	Pinto beans
Broad beans	Haricot beans	Split peas
Butter beans	Kidney beans	

Sugars and Sweeteners
Artificial sweeteners, all, including:

Aspartame   Splenda
Saccharin   Sweet'N Low

And natural sweeteners, like:

Agave nectar   Cane sugar   Dextrose
Aspartame   Chocolate, sweets,   Fructose
Beet sugar   desserts, candy, etc. Honey
Brown rice syrup   Coconut sugar   Molasses
Brown sugar   Corn syrup

Asterix indicates best choice for necessary sweeteners

*Erythritol   *Sorbitol   *Xylitol
*Licorice   *Stevia

THE CHEAT SHEET

Eats on the Left...

Grains and Pseudo-seeds
Please refer to the appendix (page 290)
if you are not losing weight as quickly as you would like.

Amaranth	Kaniwa	Teff
Buckwheat	Quinoa	

Good Proteins!
Your first 100g serving is an Eat; anything after counts as a Cheat.
Try for organic and grass-fed when you can. Always choose non-GMO
soy and soy-based products.

Beef	Pea potato protein	Soy and soy-based
Chicken	Pork (Only lean cuts	products, all,
Egg (two per	of steaks, loins)	including:
portion)	Sashimi, any kind	Edamame
Fish (wild caught is	Shellfish	Tempeh
best)	Wild game	Tofu
Hemp protein		Turkey
Pea rice protein		Quorn

Good Fats
Your first serving at your first meal is an Eat;
after that it counts as a Cheat

Almond milk (250ml)	Coconut	Goat milk (60ml)
Almond butter	Coconut milk, tinned	Hemp milk (60ml)
(1 tbsp)	(40ml)	High oleic sunflower
Almonds (6)	Coconut milk,	oil Macadamia oil
Almond oil	unsweetened	Olive oil (1 tbsp)
Avocado (⅓ of a large	(250ml)	Pumpkin seed oil
or ½ of a small-sized	Extra virgin coconut	Rice milk
avocado)	oil (1 tbsp)	Tahini (1 ½ tbsp)
Buttermilk (60ml)	Flaxseed oil	Walnut oil (1 tbsp)

Grains

Barley
Bulgur wheat
Cereal
Corn (yes, corn is not a vegetable.
  It's a grain)
Millet
Oats

Oat bran
Popcorn
Rice, all kinds
Rye
Sorghum
Spelt
Triticale

Proteins

Oysters
Liver
Veal
Duck

Fatty cuts or preparation of beef
  and pork including:
Sausage
Bacon
Ham

Fats

Butter
Corn oil
Cottonseed oil
Ghee
Grapeseed oil

Lard
Margarine
Palm oil
Peanut oil
Rapeseed oil

Safflower oil
Shortening
Soybean oil
Sunflower oil
Vegetable oil

THE CHEAT SHEET

Nuts and Nut Butters

First serving, that totals 100 calories is an Eat, after that it's a Cheat (always pick a brand free of sugar and palm oil).

Pistachios	Cashews	Hazelnuts
Peanuts	Walnuts	Pecans
Macademia	Brazil nuts	Soy nuts

Condiments and Spices

The ingredients that make vegetables taste good!

Allspice	Dried chilli pepper	Nutritional yeast
Aniseed	Fennel seed	Oregano
Basil	Fenugreek	Parsley
Bay leaves	Fish sauce	Peppercorns
Cacao	Garlic	Rosemary
Capers	Ginger	Saffron
Caraway seed	Horseradish	Sage
Cardamom	Hot sauce	Salsa
Carob	Jalapeño	Sauerkraut
Cayenne	Kimchee	Savoury
Celery seed	Lavender	Salt
Chilli flakes	Lemon	Soy (but only your
Chilli oil	Lemongrass	first serving)
Coriander	Licorice	Star anise
Cinnamon	Liquid aminos	Thyme
Cloves	Mace	Turmeric
Coriander seed	Marjoram	Vanilla
Cumin	Mint, all kinds	Vinegar, all kinds
Curry powder	Mustard	Wasabi
Dill	Nutmeg	

The list goes on and on. Take a trip to the spice section for inspiration.

and Cheats to the Right…

Nuts and Nut butters

Peanuts   Peanut butter

Condiments, Spices, Dressings and Sauces

Apple sauce   Hollandaise sauce   Steak sauce
Baba ghanoush   Hummus   Tartar sauce
Barbecue sauce   Jam   Teriyaki sauce
Bearnaise sauce   Ketchup   Soy sauce
Chutney   Marmalade   Any kind of spread
Cocktail sauce   Mayonnaise   or dip
Gravy   Peanut sauce
Hoisin sauce   Plum sauce

The Cheat Sheet is a loose framework that teaches you how to eat. Don't get hung up on calories or how you're going to do this every day. You can eat unlimited, unlimited, unlimited amounts of Eats. That's right – you are on a diet, and we are telling you that you can eat as much as you want! You can totally do this, right?

I felt that on other diets, I didn't know what I could 'safely' eat, so I restricted myself to a few very low-calorie, low-fat, low-sugar foods to rely completely on. My body was so deprived, I found myself thinking about food constantly. Now I feel that I know what better choices are and I understand that it's Ok to everything in moderation.

– Kendra S.

A common reaction when some people see the Cheat Sheet for the first time is that they say something like, "But I don't eat any of the Eats!" And that's a really big deal because they'll look at the meals and think, I have to eat salad, that's game over. But look further – you don't just eat salad on The Cheats and Eats Lifestyle Programme.

Cheat Lifestyle Programme Math

Here's what you need to keep in mind when you prepare a meal:

$$Protein + Fat + Eats = Losing Weight$$

What do we mean by that? In every meal, make sure that you have a traditional protein (chicken, fish, two eggs, or lean cuts of grass-fed beef and pork) or protein powder the size of your palm (usually a scoop or two), roughly a tablespoon of fats, and as many other Eats as you want with Cheats on top. If you focus on the unlimited Eats, we promise you will feel full. It can be anything on the Eats list: sautéed kale, artichokes, tomatoes, black beans and salsa or something like sweet potatoes sprinkled with smoked paprika. It doesn't matter what Eats you choose as long as they makes up most of your plate and that you actually eat all of them.

The list is the list – Eats are always free. But you have to limit your Cheats. However, there are always exceptions to the rule!

There are four exceptions to the Cheats. Think of them as "first-serving Eats" rather than Cheats. Your first serving of each item listed below is an Eat, then it becomes a Cheat:

1. Your first traditional protein of the day is free. A serving is usually about the size of your palm or 100g of chicken, beef, fish, two eggs or protein powder. After this first serving, they are Cheats.
2. Your first fruit of the day (other than the unlimited fruits).
3. Your first healthy fat of the day is free (one tablespoon of olive oil, half an avocado or one tablespoon of almond butter for example).
4. Your first cup of black coffee.

This is what we'd like you to do but in some cases, when you're at a place or an event where you can't – it's Ok.

And one other exception? You get to earn a cheats! If you're having one of our protein shake recipes, you earn a cheat. You can also earn other cheats during the three-week plan. More on that later.

VERY IMPORTANT: Yes, beans and the seed grains, potatoes, sweet potatoes in the eats list are unlimited. They're unlimited because they're high-nutrient foods and rich in fibre. HOWEVER: Have some sense...go with the bang-for-your-buck vegetables as your 80 per cent. If you're eating two sweet potatoes every meal and you're having trouble losing weight, or you're eating more than half a tin of beans at a meal (which may be really hard with all those greens), you're going to want to limit these.

It's really important to *not portion-control your vegetables*. Eat unlimited quantities! They are nutrient rich and bulk out the diet, which helps to keep you feeling full. You can't get too much of kale, or Swiss chard, or broccoli, or tomatoes. Forget everything you've ever heard about counting calories and portion control when it comes to vegetables – Eat them, Eat them, Eat them – **as many as you want** at every meal. It seems counter intuitive, but it's important. There is absolutely no reason to portion-control your vegetables, which is why they are unlimited on the Eats list.

A friend recently called me up and said, "Jackie, I love The Cheats and Eats Lifestyle Programme but I'm hungry on it!" so I asked her what she was eating. She said she was eating chicken breast, and spinach sautéed with olive oil and chilli flakes (one of my favourites). I asked her the size of the chicken breast, and it was about the size of a deck of cards, so I knew she was eating enough protein for satiation. Then I asked her about how much olive oil she used and she said about a spoonful, so she was getting enough fat. But then I asked about the spinach. She was only eating half of a box of frozen spinach – about 125g! No wonder she was hungry! I told her to eat the entire package the next time she made dinner and call me back. She sounded a bit sceptical, but she did what I said. Afterwards, when she called me back, she told me she was amazed by how full she felt. *And* as she continues to eat this way, the weight continues to come off!

To be really satisfied it is also crucial that you eat a source of protein and a good fat, or you'll end up hungry. Don't skip eating a source of protein with your meals as this can leave you feeling hungry. When we are hungry, we tend to make bad choices that can make us feel like we don't have the discipline to follow through on our goal of losing weight. But as we explained earlier, success really isn't about that. It's about making good decisions – which you do when you're not hungry, when you're full and satisfied. That's why The Cheats and Eats Lifestyle Programme works – because it gives your body what it needs to be satiated, and enables you to make the best choices possible.

You need protein and fat to feel full, which will help you to shed the weight. Nutrient-rich vegetables fill you up, but nobody is going to eat 1kg of vegetables at every meal, so you'll need the protein and fat. More importantly, everything we've been told time and again about portion control, fat, low-fat diets and what have you is rubbish. We have been conditioned to believe that portions of everything matter, when they don't. Only the foods that don't work in our favour, only the Cheats, need to be counted.

Apologies for being repetitive, but just to reiterate the point again: **Vegetables are the best diet pill because they have tons of nutrients, are low in calories,** *and keep you feeling full.* Even the most committed trip up sometimes, getting tired of making vegetables or sick of cooking altogether, so just grabbing whatever is in the refrigerator. I'll eat a piece of chicken and half of an avocado, but no veggies because I don't feel like making spinach or a salad. And then I'll be starving one hour later!

 I can't go for more than three days without eating kale. I think the biggest thing is the idea of stuffing myself with vegetables! No portion control on salads or vegetables in general. So, I can fill my plate with a colorful and delicious pile of veggies and get completely full, and all that nice fibre keeps me full and satisfied for a long time. Having nutrient-dense food makes *all* the difference.

So, time for some real-life example of how The Cheats and Eats Lifestyle Programme math works. Let's say that you decided to make a two-egg omelette for breakfast. The two eggs are your first traditional protein of the day, and the olive oil or butter you cook it in would be the first fat. Remember your exceptions to the rule? So, your two-egg omelette is actually Cheat free! But if you only ate two eggs, you'd be hungry. You need to add some Eats to make you full. Pile on the broccoli, mushrooms, onions, tomatoes, and fresh spinach. Maybe a little basil. And now you're really starting to add in some Eats.

If you decided to serve your omelette with a slice of toast then this is where the Cheats would come in. Each piece of bread is roughly 100 calories, which means you've used just one cheat of the 10 cheats a day you have available in the first week. Now that you've had a filling, healthy breakfast full of Eats, you will not be hungry until it's time for lunch, and you still have nine Cheats left for the day!

Does that make sense? Ultimately, the ideal Cheat Lifestyle Programme meal is made up of the same three things: a protein, a fat, and Eats – plus Cheats, if you want.

The only "rules" to cheating properly are:

+ Eat Three Meals a Day Vs. Snacking
+ Concentrate on What's Going to Make You Full – The Eats

Even though you are going to be on a diet, while you are doing The Cheats and Eats Lifestyle Programme, you will be fuller than you've ever been in your life – because you're piling on the Eats.

Why Three Meals a Day?

Snacking has become an eating habit that many people have adopted. People often freak out when they realise that they will be eating just three real meals a day on this diet. Why? Because many of us have become addicted to snacking. This method of eating does work for some people (athletes especially), but it does not help you lose weight. The theory goes that if you constantly feed your system, it "burns" calories constantly. But really, what dieticians have found is that eating small, frequent meals actually increases your appetite and the number of calories you eat, making it harder to lose weight. And though there is some benefit to constantly burning your body's engine, it simply doesn't make up for the extra calories. Three different studies – cited in *The British Journal of Nutrition*[20], *Obesity*[21], *and The American Journal of Nutrition*[22] – have shown that there are no weight-loss benefits to eating small, frequent meals.

What we'd like for you to do is eat three meals a day, and entirely avoid snacking if you can. If you have a challenging work and home schedule, or have been on a frequent eating schedule (diet or not), you may find that you are starving and have to eat a snack between meals during the first week on Cheat System. We totally get that, and it's Ok.

Another thing that we want you to try to do is to not eat during the two to three hours before you go to bed. We eat for energy so eating at that point in the day doesn't really make sense. A lot of us eat before bed as a reaction to our emotions, not because of hunger.

When we are alone with our thoughts, often we turn to food (or to alcohol) to alleviate thinking about deeper issues. That's why most of us drink wine with dinner or eat snacks while watching TV. The slight you feel because your sister chose someone else to talk to instead of you, the kid that's making your son's life hell by teasing him incessantly, your husband's inability to understand your frustrations – for all of these you may turn to cheese and chocolate or Cabernet to soothe. If you are one of those people, here are two ways to help you. First, check out the Advanced sections in the next few chapters – each has an emotional component that will help you cope. Secondly, be sure to eat plenty of Eats during the day – so you're completely full after dinner at night. It will help you say no to the ice cream your partner pulls out of the freezer at 10 p.m.

A Note About Breakfast

There are many places people make mistakes in terms of diet, but the most common is breakfast. People usually tend to fall in one of two categories: 1. They skip breakfast hoping that to "save" calories for later – which typically results in a binge later on that day; 2. They have every intention of getting a good start but end up eating dessert for breakfast: you're late to work or dropping off your kids at school, so you grab a "wholegrain" muffin and a skinny latte. No matter how healthy that sounds – even though it has the words wholegrain and skinny in it, even though you think you're making a slightly better choice – you're still eating dessert for breakfast. And unfortunately, that sets you up for a day of sugar-binge disaster.

Most people are just looking for an easy way to eat something nutritious that tastes good in the five minutes between getting ready for work and heading out the door. It's tough to make a healthy breakfast in the amount of time most of us have, but conventional breakfast food, especially what's commercially available, simply doesn't contain enough Eats. And as you know, the Eats are the diet pill that keeps you full and energised. Since most of us don't have the time to make a full breakfast with plenty of Eats, here's a solution.

In Chapter 7, we're going to teach you how to use quality ingredients to make the best meal replacement shakes. These shakes take less than five minutes to make, use ingredients that are easy to always have on hand, can satisfy your sweet tooth, give you energy and fill you up so that you won't be hungry until it's time for lunch. You won't be going through sugar withdrawal all morning from that latte and muffin, and your tummy won't grumble in your 11 a.m. meeting. And you'll lose weight. You won't believe you haven't done this before now. And you'll want to pass it along to everyone because they will be thanking you for months for turning them on to such an easy way to eat a great-tasting breakfast and lose weight!

When thinking about how your meals should be eaten throughout the day, we suggest considering switching up the size of your breakfast and dinner, or even switching the actual foods altogether. Often this depends on time and your commitment to cooking. Dinner can be a small meal like breakfast, while breakfast can be a big meal like dinner. You could have chicken for breakfast and an omelette for dinner.

Regardless of how you plan your meals, the key is to focus on the Eats. Have your "eaties" for breakfast, lunch and dinner and the "cheaties" on the side, as a condiment.

Do I Have to Be a Gourmet Chef?

Definitely, definitely not! I used to be totally intimidated by cooking. I grew up in a house where people were obsessed with food – during breakfast, we would talk about lunch; at lunch we were talking about dinner. At dinner, we were talking about what we would eat the next day. I felt like I was always talking about food. Dinner was always a big production. Everything revolved around food – if we were going somewhere, we had to figure out where we were going for lunch. By the time I became an adult, I was so completely finished with talking about eating that I completely rejected cooking and food.

I would always think, "Cooking is so much work, why can't I just grab a slice of pizza for a few dollars and move on with my day?" But today, I cook. I serve healthy meals to my family that are easy to make. And you can too, even if you are like me and don't particularly love cooking.

However, if you are already a cook, you will enjoy making the recipes on this diet, and experimenting with the recipes you already love. Many people who follow The Cheats and Eats Lifestyle Programme use the Eats list as an ingredient list and shape their recipes around an Eat, later adding in a protein, a fat and perhaps a Cheat. There's an entire section with recipes called the Cheating Gourmet later in the book.

All the foods listed in our Eats and Cheats lists can be found in any normal supermarket. The focus should be on making healthy food taste good. If you don't know the first thing about cooking – even if you don't know how to soak beans or boil an egg – this diet is for you, too.

A lot of diet experts and health gurus tell you that you should prioritise cooking, that you have to learn how to cook in order to eat a healthy diet. Whilst it is definitely useful, just because you don't enjoy cooking doesn't mean you need to be unhealthy. Grilled fish or meat with veggies or even something as simple as chicken breast cooked in a ready-made jar of tomato sauce, with veggies and brown rice works. No chef skills necessary!

We're going to give you all the things you need to succeed no matter what your abilities or willingness to cook. We've noticed that even the most reluctant cook can make one thing that tastes delicious. And when friends and family fall all over themselves saying how good it is, you think, "Well, that was easy, why don't I try another recipe?". And if the same thing happens, you start thinking "I can do this." And that's how you build your cooking muscles! Some people learn to love cooking, while others just do it because they have to. Wherever you fall on the spectrum, The Cheats and Eats Lifestyle Programme will work for you.

Frequently Asked Questions About Cheating and Eating

Sometimes after people have looked through the list and The Cheats and Eats Lifestyle Programme, then email me to ask questions about why certain foods are Eats while others are Cheats. Here are a few examples of the most commonly asked questions:

+ **Why are artificial sweeteners Cheats?**
Though these products contain very few – or even zero – calories, most may be counterproductive to losing weight. Artificial sweeteners such as Splenda, Sweet'n'Low, and Equal are considered Cheats because of the effect they may have on our eating behaviour. Statements from both Cancer Research UK and the US National Cancer Institute have

Throughout this chapter, we're going to give you Cheat Cuts: little tips and tricks fed back to us from people following The Cheats and Eats Lifestyle Programme that make eating healthy super easy. Here's the first one: Buy pre-cut and pre-washed EVERYTHING. Every supermarket sells pre-cut produce, and pre-washed salad leaves, spinach, chard and stir-fry mixes. Buy jars of salsa or tomato sauce or ready-made hummus instead of making your own (just read the label to make sure there aren't any hidden ingredients that you don't want to be eating). Anything you can get where the prep work has been done for you is well worth buying. Opening packages doesn't require nearly as much effort as becoming your own sous chef.

said that sweeteners don't cause cancer, with strong evidence that they are safe for humans. All sweeteners in the EU also undergo rigorous safety assessment before they can be used in food and drinks. Artificial sweeteners can also be useful for people with diabetes that need to watch their blood sugar levels.

Studies have however suggested that artificial sweeteners may alter your taste buds, causing you to crave sweeter and sweeter and sweeter foods in order to satisfy the "sweet tooth" you develop by using them. The downside of eating large amounts of foods and drinks sweetened this way is that may increase your energy intake and contribute to weight gain.

This is the main reason why artificial sweeteners are Cheats, eating them in excess may make it difficult for you to lose weight.

The No-Cook Cheat Lifestyle Programme Meal

You only have to do three things to have a cooking-free meal with only two Cheats!

1. Go to the supermarket and buy a frozen meal (Go for organic if you can and make sure the dinner has a traditional protein). At the same time, buy some frozen spinach, greens, or another Eat you like.

2. When you're ready to eat, remove whatever carbohydrate (rice, pasta) is included in the frozen dinner. (If you want to keep the carbohydrate, that's fine – but count it as Cheats.) Keeping a sauce is Ok, or adding your own is fine, too. Then take the frozen Eat and add it on top of the frozen dinner.

3. Heat and serve.

✦ Why is coffee considered a Cheat?

Coffee is one of our biggest addictions. The problem isn't the coffee itself, necessarily: one cup of black coffee in the morning is fine – and it may even have weight loss benefits if you choose to work out within 45 minutes of drinking it. The problem with coffee is two-fold: first, I see people drinking entire pots of coffee or excessive amounts and not losing weight; and second, most people drink it with too much cream, milk, and/or sugar – making a low-calorie drink really high in calories, and resulting in the same sugar crash as the "dessert for breakfast" example.

If you find that you want or need caffeine during the day, drink green tea. It contains powerful antioxidants called catechins that black tea and coffee do not have. These catechins are not only good for your health, but research[23] has suggested they may even help to promote fat loss (although the effect is small).

٠ In the exceptions to the rules, why are some of the Eats then Cheats considered equal when many of them have different fat, calorie and fibre content? For example, two eggs are equal to 100g of chicken and those have different nutritional profiles.

Remember, we've done the work for you and we've worked forgiveness into the plan. The focus is on the Eats, not the Cheats. So as long as we've listed something as an Eat as your first serving then as a Cheat, it's an Eat, then a Cheat.

٠ Can I "bank" my Cheats for a special occasion?

Yes you can! If you have an event on Saturday, you can have fewer cheats during the week and save them for the event. You might see the scale go up the next day after the event if you weigh yourself, but it won't be a true number until the following day when you've gone right back to your typical Eats and Cheats day.

٠ Are there any foods that aren't on the list?

No. You can eat every food, no matter what. All foods are either a Cheat or an Eat. But it's important to know that all Cheats are not equal. There are some foods we'd prefer that you reduce significantly in your diet, or avoid altogether:

- ٠ Smoked foods.
- ٠ Processed cold cuts.
- ٠ High fructose corn syrup, any sugar substitutes, and other processed chemicals. If you can't pronounce it, you shouldn't eat it. Avoid sugar, processed food, wheat, soy, corn, anything that people have manufactured that hits your satiation point (salt, sugar, and fat), anything that you can't stop eating – basically all junk food, potato chips, candy, etc. They've spent billions of dollars on marketing, advertising and chemistry labs to make those foods irresistible.
- ٠ Peanut butter. Whenever you can, swap almonds or walnuts for peanuts.
- ٠ Limit soy products, including soy milk, soy sauce, and tofu.
- ٠ An overwhelming amount of fruit (though your first fruit of the day is free).

The reason I ask you to reduce your intake of these Cheats in particular is because I want you to get results. This list was created very carefully and strategically. If you increase the amount of vegetables and decrease processed foods and chemicals you eat, your body simply runs better.

We can't say it enough: eat your Eats, especially vegetables. One thing we've learned from listening to people on The Cheats and Eats Lifestyle Programme is that there is a strong correlation between health and weight loss. Here's the secret: it takes time to get your health back in order. People abuse their bodies for 25 years and think they can go on a six-week natural health cleanse and all will be well. This is not the case. You will definitely lose your 10 pounds in three weeks but your health goals should be something you stick to, not something you fail at and then feel badly about yourself. Being on The Cheats and Eats Lifestyle Programme will get you results both in the short term for your weight and in the long term for your overall health.

As part of that, we want you to think differently about every meal. Instead of thinking, "We're having roast beef tonight; what vegetable should we have on the side?", we want you to think, "What vegetables are we having for dinner with roast beef (Cheats!) on the side?" Change how you think about sandwiches. Bread isn't necessary most of the time; you can eat chicken salad as part of a bigger green salad instead of automatically making a sandwich. Think of the Cheats as your "side" dish and the Eats as your "main".

As you start to increase your vegetable consumption you'll probably start to find that you actually eat fewer than 10 Cheats a day. Why? Because you'll be so satisfied from the high-nutrient foods you're eating from the left side of the menu that you simply won't need to eat as much from the Cheats. *The more you increase your Eats and decrease Cheats, the quicker you'll see the numbers on your scale go down.* In other words, focusing on the fact that you can eat unlimited Eats won't make you feel limited by your weekly number of Cheats.

Should I Take Any Supplements?

Supplements are a useful way to fill any shortfalls in your diet but food should always come first. Most people can benefit from a multivitamin and mineral supplement but following

The Cheats and Eats Lifestyle Programme and filling up on the eats you will get all and more than the amount vitamins and minerals required for optimal nutrient intake. If you don't eat at least one serving of oily fish each week then we recommend taking a 1000mg omega-3 supplement that contains EPA and DHA. These are also available for vegans that harness these essential anti-inflammatory fatty acids from algae. We recommend supplementing your diet with a probiotic. Gut bacteria play a key role in nutrient absorption and the synthesis of certain vitamins. Research has also shown that gut bacteria may help to reduce inflammation in the body[24] and may even be linked to appetite, obesity and mental health (although the research is in its very early stages). The balance of bacteria in your gut can be compromised by stress, bad diet and medication. Look for a supplement that contains trains of Lactobacillus and Bifidobacterium and at least 20 billion bacteria per dose.

It's important to pick your supplements wisely and there is no benefit to chucking back handfuls of supplements when they are not required. Look for a trusted brand whose supplements are GMP approved, which is the gold standard for good practice and quality. Our preferred brand is Healthspan (www.healthspan.co.uk)

Will This Work for Guys?

Yes. If you're a big guy and are very active you may find yourself adding a few Cheats if you're still hungry eating only 10 per day. With extra Cheats, the scale may move a bit slower, but you'll have to test it out and figure out what works best for your body and energy level. Some men find that when they are in the groove, they eat less than 10 Cheats on most days because their staples are Eats: sweet potatoes, beans, vegetables, seeds, nuts and various soups. This is what gives great energy all day, and keeps even "insane man hunger" satisfied. If you're an athlete, please go to page 290 in the appendix for more information about The Cheats and Eats Lifestyle Programme for athletes.

Cheating and Eating Out

Here's the truth about Cheat System, from someone who's actually been on it and been successful: I don't say no to anything, and you shouldn't, either. **You should feel free to use Cheats as you want to.** You can save up Cheats over the course of a day or even the course of a week and splurge on a particular meal, or you can use a Cheat or two at every meal. Personally, I find it easier to use Cheats in bunches because it's easier to keep track of that way – but you should do what works for you.

For example, you can save your Cheats up for a special occasion or happy hour. If you're eating the Eats most of the time, your body or weight won't be all that affected by one happy hour or meal out. I go many days using only six Cheats per day because I'm eating the Eats and feel full. I save up Cheats so that I can go crazy when I am eating out every once in a while. On those occasions, I enjoy anything I want and I don't gain weight.

I really enjoy that on The Cheats and Eats Lifestyle Programme because there is nothing that you can't eat. You can eat any 'bad' or 'unhealthy' food as long as it's in moderation. Somehow, knowing that helps me have more motivation to eat good foods."
– Sara

Eating out is actually why I developed The Cheats and Eats Lifestyle Programme the way I did. You don't have to stress out at a restaurant and worry about preparation, fat, fibre or calories. You just have to know what is a Cheat and how many of them you have. You don't have to stop going out to eat with your friends, you don't have to mentally prepare for dinner with your spouse, or try to be psychologically strong around your co-workers when they invite you out to celebrate someone's promotion.

Guard Your Mind

Losing weight is not whether we're capable of being psychologically strong; we are. But we all need flexibility in our lives. People are complicated and contradictory – it's just part of human nature. On The Cheats and Eats Lifestyle Programme, we accept that. We stop beating ourselves up for eating chocolate or chips. The fact is you're going to eat cheese and crackers once in a while, but it's not the end of the world and you can still lose weight!

It's important not to put yourself under too much pressure. You have done the hardest part by committing to lose weight and The Cheats and Eats Lifestyle Programme is here to help you, not challenge you to do that. If it all goes wrong and you just have one of those days where it all goes completely off-plan, then don't ever see this as a failure or reason to give up and fall into old habits. Focus on what you have achieved so far and just pick up where you left off the following day.

The Cheat Sheet and The Cheats and Eats Lifestyle Programme are designed to work in real life by teaching you to accept the fact that you're going to make mistakes and that even if you cheat on your diet, you will still lose weight.

It's very easy to eat out and be social on this diet: wherever you go, you just need to estimate what the Cheats are. Look at your plate: other than a palm-sized portion of protein, a cherry tomato of fat, and all of your Lats and everything else is a Cheat. As you get more familiar with counting your Cheats, you'll have a rough notion of how many Cheats something is. For example, a slice of bread is usually around one Cheat. A restaurant serving of pasta, especially with the sauce is usually five or six Cheats.

When you're eating out, you can use your knowledge of Eats and Cheats to help you order. There is always the option of a grilled piece of fish or meat with vegetables and you can request any sauces on the side. Perhaps you really want a burger? Well order it without the bun or give up your fries for an extra serving of salad. You can also stick to ordering two starters if that works.

Eating out is a luxury for most people so you should allow yourself to indulge a little but if you are trying to stick with The Cheats and Eats Lifestyle Programme then don't make things difficult for yourself. Don't be fooled into thinking you're going to order something and only eat half of it because more often than not, you won't. Don't agree to share several puddings with the table if you know you're just going to keep picking at every dessert. You could always settle for a green tea or learn to pick your pleasure (see below) to help you to manage social occasions when following The Cheats and Eats Lifestyle Programme.

Pick Your Pleasure: Wine, Bread or Dessert

When you go out to eat, you're not going to have just a little bit of bread, or a little bit of wine, or a little bit of dessert. If you go crazy once in a while that's Ok, but if you're someone who ends up eating out more than you'd like you need to know how to handle it.

Your pleasure, whether it's wine, bread or dessert, will still be a Cheat. But going a little overboard on one is certainly better than going overboard on all three. Personally, I tend to pick wine or the dessert because bread just isn't worth it for me. But what you pick is up to you.

We decided on the "pick your pleasure" idea because many people have their own little rules such as the three-bite rule at dessert (you could order any dessert you want but you could only have three bites). However, for most of us, once you taste the delicious dessert it's more than likely you're going to eat the whole thing, period. This way, you only go overboard on one thing – and not everything.

Be mindful

Understanding what to eat is one thing but how you eat may play a part in your ability to lose weight. How many of us eat without thinking or do not set time aside for meals, instead choosing to wolf down our food on the run between meetings or sat at our computer whilst trying to meet a deadline? Modern lifestyles influence the way we eat and can encourage weight gain, indigestion, anxiety and other negative food-related behaviours as well as leaving us unable to identify when we are hungry or full. Eating mindfully not only allows you to enjoy and appreciate your food but gives your brain a chance to register that you have eaten, which helps with fullness. The concept is about paying full attention to your experiences, cravings and physical cues when eating.

Mindful eating is simple and makes common sense but many of us have got wrapped up in our busy schedules and often view food a necessity rather than a pleasure and opportunity to take time out for yourself during the day. Try and adopt these simple practical techniques to help you to apply a little mindfulness to the way you eat:

+ Serve your food on a plate and sit down to eat without distraction.
+ Chew your food slowly and put your cutlery down between mouthfuls.
+ Assess your hunger and satiety.
+ Savour your food and enjoy every texture and flavour it has to offer.

Research has suggested that mindfulness may help with stress eating and reduce cortisol levels, which may in turn help to reduce belly fat over time[25]. The Cheats and Eats Lifestyle Programme is about including the foods you take pleasure from eating so apply a little mindfulness to savour every mouthful and make the most out of mealtimes.

This Is not 'Diet' Food

I want you to stop eating "substitution foods". What I mean by that is eating a turkey burger and sweet potato fries when you really want a burger and fries, or substituting some kind of weird health-food pizza with brown-rice crust or wholewheat crust for a normal pie. All of those concoctions – and they are concoctions – don't replace the emotional yummy taste you're going for. Often once you're done with its substitution, you're going to still want the pizza or the burger – and then you've doubled the calories of that craving! Save your Cheats for things you really want, not for poor substitutes. The trend of "let's have quinoa pizza" rarely works because it tastes like cardboard and you still want real pizza after anyway.

Change the focus to the Eats. Substituting "healthy" concoctions for what you really want isn't satisfying. Figuring out which artificial sweetener might be better for you is a waste of time. Sure, some natural sweeteners such as honey may be viewed as being better than others but at the end of the day, it doesn't matter because it's all sugar, it all lacks micronutrients, and it's all Cheats.

 Honestly, The Cheats and Eats Lifestyle Programme is the best thing you have given me so far. I followed it very extensively for a month and now it has become a template for how I eat. It helped me plan for when I wanted something sweet. It was really easy to determine how many calories I was really consuming and where to make allowances for treats. It made it so easy and now no food has to be off limits. It gave me choices but still keeps me in control of where I like to be.

The Cheats and Eats Lifestyle Programme has helped thousands of people to lose weight and in the next three chapters you will find the meal plans and recipes for the next 21 days that are going to change the way you eat, how you feel and what size you wear. What you'll learn in those chapters will help you lose up to a stone in just three weeks!

CHAPTER 5

The Cheats and Eats Lifestyle Programme Week One

Eat the Eats, and You Have 10 Cheats

This week, we want you to focus on the Eats. Try to incorporate as many as you can. Eat as many Eats as you want; Eats are unlimited! If you're still hungry when you finish your first plate of Eats, go for a second!

Calories are not created equal. One hundred calories of broccoli are going to provide you with much more nutrition than the same amount of sugar. The nutrients in the Eats from the Cheat Sheet will give you the nutrients you need to stay satiated and full until your next meal. That's the reason those Eats are completely unlimited. The portions for the traditional protein (about the size of a deck of cards or of your palm) and the fat (a tablespoon or a cherry-tomato-sized dollop) are somewhat set because those aren't strictly nutrient based.

Your body will use the high micronutrients in the food you eat – it's what we call "eating for energy." If you eat The Cheats and Eats Lifestyle Programme way, you'll maintain energy levels for hours afterwards, because your body's levels of cortisol and blood sugar are completely stable. Every meal will also supply you with a rich source of micronutrients to nourish your body and keep it functioning properly. With renewed energy and optimum micronutrient intake you'll be amazed at how you feel. I did not really understand myself how eating for energy and for my body worked until I began having a high-nutrient lifestyle and started being conscious of Cheats. I avoided being tired at 11 a.m. and 2 p.m. – I had energy all day, to do the things I needed to do. The change in what I was eating made all the difference.

Remember, the **10 Cheats** you can eat every day this week are there for a reason. First, you're going to need to cheat because your body and your mind will want the Cheats. And you'll lose weight even while eating that many Cheats each day this week.

Whilst The Cheats and Eats Lifestyle Programme allows you to eat what you want, there are still boundaries and if you eat more than the Cheats allotted for each day, or the week, then this will not work – you can't cheat all the time and lose weight, period. Before you check out our sample meal plans, keep these four things in mind:

1. Get rid of your junk.
Take the issue of discipline or of willpower out of the picture. Clear your kitchen of temptation and chuck the junk. You can't eat what you don't have in your home.

2. When in doubt:
Vegetables + Protein + Healthy Fats = Lose Weight
When you're thinking about what to eat at any time of the day, this should be your guide. Remember what a Cheats and Eats meal looks like: a palm-sized portion of traditional protein, a tablespoon portion of healthy fat and at least a grapefruit-sized portion of vegetables – and as many additional vegetables as you want (and Cheats on top!)

3. You don't have to *make* anything!
Don't feel like cooking? Not up for washing lettuce? You can use the Cheat Sheet to create something. A can of tuna with a bag of ready prepared salad, chopped herbs, tinned white beans and dressed with olive oil and lemon juice is a nutritious meal that requires zero effort. Don't worry about recipes if cooking isn't your thing. I often put together the strangest combinations because it's easy and it's what appealed to me at the moment.

4. If you do cook, rotating through meals you love is fine!
Eating The Cheats and Eats Lifestyle Programme way should not feel like prison. Find three or four meals that you love, savour and look forward to and are psyched about. This week, I want you to focus on finding these three or four meals that taste good and give you energy. Put them into standard rotation, and make them meals you can rely on to satisfy you in a healthy way. When you feel like experimenting you can – but these will be your 'go-to' dishes.

5. Include at least one serving of oily fish each week.
We introduced you to the effects of inflammation in the previous chapters and getting a good supply of omega-3 fatty acids in your diet is essential. Oily fish are the richest source and include fresh salmon, trout, tuna, mackerel, herring as well as tinned anchovies and salmon. If you don't eat oily fish then take a daily 1000mg omega-3 supplement that contains both EPA and DHA. Vegan omega-3 supplements source these fatty acids from sea algae.

Focus on the Eats, But...

Remember that diet is only 75 per cent of what goes into the losing weight – and the other 25 per cent comes from getting your body moving. So, remember what Nicola discussed in Chapter 3: Your base point is to try and walk 10,0000 steps every day. But it doesn't have to be all at once; you can get off the bus and walk half the way to work, use the stairs at work, take the dog out for a walk in the evening or clean the house. It doesn't matter how you do it, just make sure that you move! This isn't a HIIT class but a small change you can make and stick to will provide some consistency in the way you introduce activity into your daily life. If you currently do not exercise then work on getting from zero to one rather than straight to 10.

Tracking Your Success

These days you're not on your own when it comes to making informed decisions about diet and exercise. Wearable tech – a name that covers a range of device such as smart watches, activity trackers and even smart clothing – is becoming more prevalent. So too is the range of smartphone apps available, many of which work in conjunction with wearable tech. Together they can track your activity, calculate your burned calories, help you keep a food diary, monitor your heart rate and even create exercise programmes for you.

Several studies have shown that people who keep food diaries are more likely to succeed at losing weight and there is some evidence to suggest that tracking steps keeps you motivated towards your activity goals.

As wearable tech, apps and at-home testing of things like DNA and microbiome advance, the future is going to entail more personalised approaches to nutrition and exercise. In the future one size is unlikely to fit all.

Healthspan have just launched their NutriCoach well-being platform. At the heart is an app that links to Healthspan's own activity tracker (it can also take data from other popular trackers or apps like Fitbit or Apple Healthkit) and a smart body composition scale (that provides not just weight but measures things such as body fat and muscle mass). The Healthspan app allows comprehensive food logging, provides a daily health score and, in conjunction with your activity tracker, logs your motion and calories burned. After answering a few simple questions, and as your data develops over time, the app will also generate personalised lifestyle recommendations and even allow you to tailor supplements (protein, multivitamin and electrolyte) to meet your needs.

Keeping track of what you eat and what you do rules out the possibility of kidding yourself. If things aren't moving in the right direction you've got everything logged, which is useful if you need to make some changes and particularly useful when it comes to consuming the right variations of nutrients for your body. Think back to the last time you told yourself you deserved a cookie (or any treat) because you'd been on a half-an-hour run. No one can argue with that – of course you deserved it.

Cheat Week One Meal Plan

This is going to be easy. We don't want you to get hung up on what the meal plans here look like. What we do want you to get hung up on is that unless you eat from the Eats category, you're limited to 1,000 calories of Cheats per day and no one can survive on that. You must eat your Eats.

Treat the meal plans as guidance and inspiration, not as rules to follow. Feel free to mix and match. These are simply meant to show you how Cheating and Eating works in practise. You can find all of our recipes in Chapter 9, starting on page 144.

Week One Meal Plan

Day 1

BREAKFAST: 2 eggs scrambled with 1 slice bacon, mushroom and spinach, half a grapefruit, herbal or green tea, or one cup of black coffee

Total Cheats: 1 – from the bacon; remember, your first serving of protein here is free

LUNCH: Weight Loss Short cut Soup (2 servings) with Easy Foil Rosemary Chicken (100g); bring a Thermos!

Total Cheats: 3 – from the coconut milk (2) and chicken (1)

IF EATING OUT: Chipotle Bowl with palm-size chicken, pico de gallo and salsa, palm-size beans, golf ball-size portion of guacamole

Total Cheats: 3 – from the chicken (2) and guacamole (1)

DINNER: Hot Italian Salmon Garlic Scampi with lots of romaine and Caesar salad dressing, 125ml glass of wine

Total Cheats: 4.5 – 2 tablespoons of the salad dressing (1), salmon (2), and wine (1.5)

Cheats: You've used eight Cheats. You have two remaining.

Day 2

BREAKFAST: Chocolate Almond Sea Salt Shake. You may also add 150ml–200ml of black coffee to this shake if you're having trouble giving up the sugar or cream in the coffee.

Total Cheats: 0 (Free! Because of the exceptions to the Cheat rule.)

LUNCH: Di's Hot Sausage Spice Soup (1 Portion, 1 Cheat) and Savoury Rosemary Chicken Salad

Total Cheats: 3 – from the sausage, chicken, avocado, and oil

DINNER: Prawn Taco Wraps with Black Beans and Salsa
(2 servings)
Total Cheats: 3 – from the shrimp and avocado

Cheats: You've used six Cheats. You have four remaining.

Day 3
BREAKFAST: Scott's Summer Breakfast Salad with 2 hard
boiled eggs, 1 cup of hot tea or 1 cup of coffee
*Total Cheats: 0 – your first protein, piece of fruit, healthy fat and
cup of coffee is free!*
LUNCH: Avocado and Bacon Chicken Salad on a large bed of
mixed greens
Total Cheats: 3 – from the chicken and cheat confetti

IF EATING OUT: Subway Grilled Chicken Salad with 1 slice
of bacon – load up on the greens! Balsamic vinaigrette
(1 tablespoon)
Total Cheats: 3 – from the chicken and dressing

SNACK: Apple with ½ tablespoon almond butter, 1 cup of
green tea
Total Cheats: 2 – from the apple and almond butter
DINNER: Spring Fresh Cherry Tomato appetiser, Insane Man
Hunger Chilli (2 servings)
Total Cheats: 3 – from the oil and beef

Cheats: You've used eight Cheats. You have two remaining.

Day 4
BREAKFAST: Brian Rigby's Mint Chocolate Chip Cookie
Smoothie
*Total Cheats: 0 – This is an approved shake and your
first serving!*

LUNCH: Boulder Athletic Recovery Salad *Total Cheats: 2*

IF EATING OUT: Large bed of mixed greens, 1 tablespoon of olive oil and freshly squeezed lemon, 100g (pack of cards sized) of whatever grilled protein is available at the restaurant
Total Cheats: (2) from the chicken and dressing

DINNER: Brian's Sweet Potato and Coconut Meatballs with Tomato Sauce (1 serving, 2 Cheats); Garlicky mashed "potatoes" (1); Roasted Broccoli with Cheat Confetti Parmesan Crisps (1.5); Pumpkin Pie (1)
Total Cheats: 5.5

Cheats: You've used seven and a half Cheats. You have two and half remaining!

Day 5
BREAKFAST: Triple Berry Smoothie (or a shake from the breakfast recipe section)
Total Cheats: 0 – This is an approved shake

LUNCH: Slow cooker Chicken and Spinach Soup; Perfect Sweet Potato Fries
Total Cheats: 3 – from the bacon, coconut milk and chicken

DINNER: Spicy Thai Curry (2 servings with a cup of rice) (3 cheats); 125ml glass of wine or 1.5 cheat worth of dark chocolate (30g or 2½ large squares)
Total Cheats: 4.5

Cheats: You've used seven and a half Cheats. You have two and half remaining.

Day 6
BREAKFAST: Chocolate Raspberry Torte Shake
Total Cheats: 0!

LUNCH: Tex-Mex Salad with crisps
Total Cheats: 2.5 – from the avocado and crisps

DINNER: Warm Cream of Tomato Soup and Classic Italian Grilled Cheese (5 Cheats); Simple Sautéed Spinach; Garlicky Mashed potatoes (1)
Total Cheats: 6 – from the coconut milk, bread, butter, cheese and avocado

Cheats: You've used eight and half Cheats. You have one and half remaining.

Day 7
BREAKFAST: Meg's Mexican Breakfast Frying pan (2 Cheats)
Total Cheats: 0 (first protein and fat are free!)

LUNCH: Italian Goddess Chicken or 100g of oily fish, a lean cut of chicken or grass-fed beef (1.5 Cheats); The Famous Puréed Energy Soup (1 serving) (1 Cheat)
Total Cheats: 2.5

DINNER: Chicken Artichoke, Mushroom, Parmesan Casserole (2 Cheats); Brussels Sprouts with Bacon (1 Cheat)
Total Cheats: 3 – from the chicken, parmesan, oil, and bacon

Cheats: You've used five and half Cheats. You have four and a half remaining.

Remember, you don't have to "cook" and make all of these recipes – you can put a few recipes into rotation instead. I only cook a couple of days a week but I know my plate. Your plate should look like:

  ◆ A 100g serving of traditional protein or plant protein
  ◆ 1 tablespoon of a healthy fat
  ◆ Tons of Eats! Fill your plate! Fill it again!
  ◆ And the rest are Cheats.

The Cheat Incentives

Each week, we'll challenge you to do a mental and a physical activity. These aren't hard but what we're asking, might be out of your comfort zone. But try each and every one – not just because you earn free Cheats, but because these are proven to help you lose more weight.

The Week One Cheat Incentives are:

- You can earn **one extra Cheat this week** if you follow The Cheats and Eats Lifestyle Programme Exercise Plan (see next page) for Week One, try a new sport or participate in an activity you loved as a child.

- You can earn **two extra Cheats this week** by taking care of actions you have been putting off. These could be little things, like fixing something broken in your home, or big things like telling a friend that she hurt your feelings. Write each action down on a list and when you're done, cross it off. The list can be handwritten, on your computer, or in the notes section on your phone (which is what I do). It just has to be somewhere outside your own thoughts. When you're done with each action – and not before – you earn one cheat for the week. (If you complete both actions, you earn two.)

Week One To Do

- Weigh yourself and record your weight. Weigh yourself at least once a week. You can't finish the marathon if you don't know where your start line is.
- Include your goal. It doesn't matter what your goal is, make sure you have one and write it down.

Week One Exercise Plan

- Complete Week One of the Cheat Lifestyle Programme Fitness Plan.
- How many daily steps are you completing on average? Look to increase this by 2000 steps a day.
- Aim to complete 30 minutes of walking a day. This can be broken down into three 10-minute walks.
- Try and opt for the more active life choice! Take the stairs not the escalator, wash the car, or sweep the garden!

CHAPTER 6

The Cheats and Eats Lifestyle Programme Week Two

Eat the Eats and Earn More Cheats

By now, you should be getting used to how cheating and eating works. This week, we're going to ask you to keep eating your Eats but limit your Cheats to eight instead of 10. So, each day this week, you will be able to eat **eight** Cheats – *but you* have an opportunity to earn **two more** each day this week through both the mental and physical Cheat incentives (at the end of this chapter), but also through eating seeds and greens. So what do you have to eat to get those extra Cheats?

1. Get a half extra cheat each day by eating a one tablespoon serving of flax or chia seeds

Though chia and flaxseeds come from different plants, both have huge health benefits. Full of protein, fibre and a useful source of omega-3 "healthy" fat, these small seeds are nutritional powerhouses, keeping you full and fighting inflammation. Both chia and flaxseeds are great in shakes, but make sure to add these last to a shake, so the mixture doesn't get thick. You can also sprinkle them over salads and soups.

2. Get one full extra Cheat each day by eating an extra 225g of greens after 5 p.m.

(A quick reminder of "greens": kale, spinach, broccoli, cabbage, mustard greens, romaine lettuce, mixed greens, Swiss chard, rocket. Check the Cheat Sheet for more.)

Remember you can only earn one and half Cheats total each day. So, you can't eat chia and flax for every meal in order to get six extra Cheats; that's not how it works (although if you want to eat that much chia and flax, good for you). It simply means that if you do either of those two things – or eat extra greens in the evening – you'll get one Cheat – and if you have the chia, you will earn an extra half Cheat each day.

I recently saw a message on our Facebook wall that said, "How could a half a pound of vegetables negate the chocolate I wanted?" I asked our Facebook friend what she meant, and whether she ate the half pound (450g) of vegetables. She had – she ate a half a pound of spinach, some broccoli, a serving of cod, and a glass of wine. But by eating the extra greens she earned an extra Cheat – she could have a one Cheat-sized portion of chocolate if she had wanted. But she didn't – because she was full!

And that's the reason it's the incentive for the week. Greens are the best diet pill available, and will make more impact on your weight than any cheat you "earn" by eating it. Remember the three stomachs from Dr. Joel Fuhrman in Chapter 2? This person is the perfect example of this concept – she ate so many greens she was completely full and couldn't even eat her Cheat if she wanted to. Of course, she can eat it another time, and that's fine, too!

Week Two Cheat Cut:
Use a food processor to chop greens up into a "green tapenade." It almost seems like you've chopped tons of herbs in your salad. It's a great way to add the extra 450g of greens to earn the extra cheat each day! You can put it on top of salads, in soups, or warm it up and put it on top of your traditional protein.

In this week's meal plan, you'll notice recipes for our soups and shakes. All are easy to make, and we want you to make one of each this week.

The shakes are a meal on their own, but if you choose to make a soup, pair it with a traditional protein for a full meal. If a soup seems intimidating to you, try making a shake – it only takes a few minutes.

Cheat Week Two Meal Plan

+ Eat your Eats, you have eight Cheats
+ Include one serving of oily fish in the week or take a 1000mg omega-3 supplement daily
+ Can earn a half extra Cheat for eating a serving chia or flaxseeds
+ Can earn one extra Cheat for eating 225g of greens after 5 p.m.
+ Try a shake or a soup this week

Remember, following the meal plans are optional. Feel free to mix and match recipes from this meal plan with what's in Chapter 9. If all you want to do one night is add some greens to a frozen dinner, that can be a great cheat free meal!

Week Two Meal Plan

Day 1

BREAKFAST: Chocolate Decadence Shake with a cup of black coffee
Total Cheats: 0 cheats!

LUNCH: Creamy Chicken salad with ⅓ of avocado 1 tablespoon of Chia Seeds (the seeds are optional, but you'll earn an extra ½ cheat if you do! 5 handfuls of chopped mixed greens; sliced tomato sprinkled with sea salt
Total Cheats: 2.5 (only 2 if you used chia)

DINNER: Tangy Tenderloin (3 cheats); Sweet Potato with cinnamon; 450g of sautéed spinach (extra cheat for the extra 450g!)
Total Cheats: Only 2 if you actually make the 900g of spinach, 3 if not.

This might seem weird, but Swiss chard and spinach are the perfect ingredients to add to our shakes! Neither changes the taste of a recipe at all and both provide nutrients you need to feel full. And remember, you earn an extra Cheat.

DESSERT: Pumpkin Pie
Total Cheats: 1 – from the sugar and coconut oil

Cheats: You've used four Cheats. You have four remaining if you followed the incentives. If not, you've used five and half cheats and you have two and half remaining.

Day 2
BREAKFAST: Mango Lassi Shake
Total Cheats: 0!

LUNCH: Tequila-Pineapple Dressing on mixed greens (0.5 Cheats); Mexican City Chicken Salad with ½ cup of black beans (1.5 Cheats)
Total Cheats: 2 – from the pineapple, avocado and chicken

DINNER: Mint and Shallot Halibut with Kale and Oven-Roasted Tomatoes (or large salad with extra kale on the side)
Total Cheats: 1.5 – from the halibut and oil

COCKTAIL: Muscle Recovery Margaritas (Or Virgin!)
Total Cheats: 2 – from the tequila

Cheats: If you had the margarita, you've used five and half Cheats and have two and half remaining; if you didn't have the margarita, you only used three and a half Cheats and have four and a half remaining.

Day 3
BREAKFAST: Leftover halibut with the Power Workout Breakfast for a powerful day! or a simple 2 egg omelette with your favourite vegetables
Total Cheats: 0!

LUNCH: Chicken with Peruvian Green Sauce (2 Cheats) Large mixed greens with Green Tea, Poppy Seed and Mint Vinaigrette (1 Cheat)
Total Cheats: 3 – from the chicken, oil, and orange juice

DINNER: Easy Italian Herb Baked Turkey (1 Cheats); The Famous Puréed Energy Soup (1 Cheat)
Total Cheats: 2 – from the meat and coconut milk

DESSERT: Easiest Apple Cinnamon Dessert (apple cored with honey and ½ teaspoon of butter and a dash of cinnamon. Microwave for 60 seconds.)
Total Cheats: 1 (your first fruit is free!)

Cheats: You've used six Cheats for the day. You have two remaining! (Three if you had the full 900g of sautéed Swiss chard.)

Day 4
BREAKFAST: Two simple hard-boiled eggs ½ sliced tomato and cucumber or fresh berries; ½ of a grapefruit; 1 cup of black coffee
Total Cheats: 0!

LUNCH: Spinach salad with watermelon, mint and caper dressing (0 Cheats) and 1 tablespoon of chia seeds; Orr's Island Vegetable Soup (0 Cheat); 100g of simple chicken breast (1.5 cheats)
Total Cheats: 2.5 (2 if you used the chia seeds)

DINNER: Cheat-Free Stir-fry with prawn or grass-fed beef
Total Cheats: 2 – from the meat and oil

Cheats: You've only used four and a half Cheats (only four if had chia seeds). You have three and a half remaining.

Day 5
BREAKFAST: Anti-inflammatory shake; Bowl of fresh berries; 1 cup of black coffee
Total Cheats: 0

LUNCH: The Basalt; simple salad of mixed greens with Magic Lime Dressing
Total Cheats: 2.5 – from the bacon and salmon

DINNER: Favourite Roast Chicken with Cheat Confetti Parmesan Crisps or Philly Cheesesteak soup; large salad, French Dijon dressing with Cheat Confetti Parmesan Crisps
Total Cheats: 3 – from the meat, oil, and cheese

Cheats: You've used five and a half Cheats but you have two and a half remaining.

Day 6
BREAKFAST: Eggs "Benedict": 2 poached eggs with 1 slice of bacon and 300g of sautéed spinach
Total Cheats: 0 (first protein, fat is free!)

LUNCH: Za'atar Grilled Chicken Strips with Warm Applewood Bacon Soup or Di's Lentil Soup
Total Cheats: 1.5 – from the chicken and oil

DINNER: Slow Cooker Fire-Roasted Tomato Beef Chilli (2 servings); 450g broccoli with Cheat Confetti Parmesan Crisps
Total Cheats: 5 – if you eat the full 900g, only 4 cheats

Cheats: You've used six and a half Cheats or five and a half if you ate the full 900g of broccoli.! You have one and half remaining!

Day 7
Breakfast: Orange Creamsicle Shake
Total Cheats: 0!

Lunch: The Famous Puréed Energy Soup or Weight Loss Short cut soup or the Carrot Ginger Soup with Brian's Sweet Potato and Coconut Meatballs
Total Cheats: 3 – from the coconut, coconut milk, and meat

Dinner: Tasty Harissa Chicken with black beans (2 Cheats; Simple Sautéed Spinach recipe
Total Cheats: 2 – from the chicken and oil

Cheats: You've used five Cheats. You have three remaining!

The Cheat Incentives

In addition to the Cheats you can earn by eating 225g of greens after 5 p.m., or by eating chia and flaxseeds, there is one more way you can earn extra Cheats this week.

The Cheat Incentive for Week Two is:

You can earn **two extra Cheats for the week** when you put an alarm in your phone that has a positive message related to your goal, or a reminder of something that makes you really happy. Your alarm could be a mantra (my "alarm" is "This is the Year") or a goal such as "150 is almost here". This trick brings your mental focus back to your goal and helps keep you on track. When focus and goals are married together, we can achieve things so much more quickly. Set the alarm to go off once or even twice a day, at different times. (If for whatever reason, adding this to your phone doesn't work for you, putting it as the background or screensaver on your computer screen or writing it down and taping that note to your mirror will work, too.)

Week Two To Do

+ Be sure to weigh yourself at least once a week.
+ Read your goal and see if it's changed. If so, choose another!

Week Two Exercise Plan

+ Complete Week Two of the Cheat Lifestyle Programme Fitness Plan.
+ Aim to complete 30 minutes of walking a day. This can be broken down into two 15-minute walks.
+ Get your dancing shoes on! Dancing is a great calorie burner. Pop on your favourite song and dance around your living room like no one is watching!

CHAPTER 7

The Cheats and Eats Lifestyle
Programme Week Three

Eat the Eats, Learn to Cheat

By this point in The Cheats and Eats Lifestyle Programme, you are enjoying the Eats more than you thought you would – and have incorporated some of our soup, shake and recipes into your everyday life. We may have gotten frustrating at some point to read, over and over again, that vegetables make you feel full because you might not have felt full every time you ate. You might still want a packet of cheese or bacon with your breakfast. But you have only been eating The Cheats and Eats Lifestyle Programme way for two weeks and sometimes your body takes time to adjust. We've noticed that all of our readers who try The Cheats and Eats Lifestyle Programme way of eating experience a transition period and you're still in the beginning phase.

There will be a moment – and if it hasn't happened yet, it will soon – where you are open to trying everything in the produce aisle because you've begun to draw connections between how fresh foods such as salad and processed foods like pizza affect how your body feels. Your body starts to link the good feeling between healthy foods and feeling bad when you eat unhealthy foods so the choice is easy. You will be shocked when you crave a salad and pass up the pizza.

You also have noticed that your taste buds are starting to change. You may be noticing that foods taste sweeter or richer, or that your palate can detect any hint of sugar or sweetness. (If you chose a rich dessert as a Cheat, you definitely know what we mean!)

This is natural; the change happens nearly every time people try The Cheats and Eats Lifestyle Programme. In addition to your palate changing, eating The Cheats and Eats Lifestyle Programme way will help you figure out what Cheats are worth it for you, and which foods you don't want to waste Cheats on. Personally, for me, it's easy to pass up bread so I can have bacon. In addition to realising what Cheats you really love, you'll begin to notice which foods you may have been binging on that stopped you from losing weight before.

Perhaps you've fallen off the wagon, and ended up gorging on cookies one night or splurged and had a margarita that turned into four with your friends. In those instances, it's really important to remember not to be hard on yourself. Don't beat yourself up over a cookie or a great night out with your friends.

Because the second you start beating yourself up, you'll go backwards. The Cheats and Eats Lifestyle Programme is designed to help you get over those little bumps in the road without turning into the type of person we all were at some point. The person who read everything about how to lose weight but didn't take any action. The person who decided to go on a diet but gave up because it was too overwhelming. The person who has a fridge full of produce but ends up ordering a takeaway.

So, if you tussled with a packet of crisps, you shouldn't worry! Pick yourself up, dust yourself off, and get back to eating your Eats. You haven't failed, you haven't lost, and you're definitely still in the game. Get back to eating your Eats – and if you want a cookie for one of your Cheats, have one!

In Week Three we'd like you to go to six Cheats. Week Three offers a few incentives to **earn another cheat for the week – by adding garlic, cinnamon, ginger or turmeric in at least one meal.** If this sounds intimidating, you don't have to do it! But if you want to earn that Cheat, adding spices into meals is a relatively easy thing to do and can transform the taste of a meal.

Cinnamon is easy to add to shakes and soups; using ginger is an easy way to flavour stir-fries, and it's surprisingly delicious on fish like salmon. Turmeric is used in a lot of cuisines. I put ginger in my tea. I sprinkle cinnamon on my sweet potato.

Some of the recipes in this week's meal plan include ginger, turmeric and cinnamon, but really if you are adventurous, the possibilities are endless. The rules from last week still applies: you can still earn an extra cheat for eating a 225g of greens after 5 p.m., or ½ a Cheat by eating chia or flax. But you can still only earn two extra Cheats each day.

Cheat Week Three Meal Plan

+ Eat your Eats, you have six Cheats per day
+ Include one serving of oily fish in the week or take a 1000mg omega-3 supplement daily
+ Earn one extra Cheat for eating 225g of greens after 5 p.m.
+ Earn ½ extra Cheat this week for eating chia or flaxseeds
+ Earn ½ extra Cheat if you add cinnamon, ginger or turmeric in one of your meals each day

Week Three Meal Plan

Day 1
BREAKFAST: 45g pinhead oats (1.5 Cheats) with 1 large chicken sausage (1.5 Cheat); mixed with mushrooms, onions and sautéed spinach (egg-less omelette!)
Total Cheats: 1.5 – from the oats (first protein free)

LUNCH: Creamy Chicken Salad (2 cheat) atop power greens (mix of kale, mustard greens and mixed greens)
Total Cheats: 1.5 – from the chicken and yogurt

DINNER: Night Eater's Best Friend Salad (2.5 Cheats); 6 almonds (0.5 cheat); 1 cup of tea
Total Cheats: 2.5 (first healthy fat is free!)

Cheats: You've used four and a half Cheats. You have one and a half remaining!

Day 2
Breakfast: Chocolate Decadence Shake
Total Cheats: 0! Your first protein and healthy fat is free.

Lunch: Carrot Ginger Soup or Butternut Squash Soup with
Za'atar Grilled Chicken Strips or whatever spice you like!
Total Cheats: 2.5 – from the coconut milk, oil and chicken

Snack: 1 apple
Total Cheats: 0 (first fruit free!)

Dinner: 100g grass-fed steak (1.5 Cheats); 1 sweet potato;
Large green salad with Simple French Dijon Dressing or
roasted asparagus (1 Cheat); 125ml glass of wine (1 Cheat)
Total Cheats: 3.5 (from the steak and the wine)

Cheats: You've used six Cheats. You have none remaining.

Day 3
Breakfast: Chocolove Shake (1.5 Cheats); 1 cup of coffee
Total Cheats: 0

Lunch: Cheat-Free Stir-fry with salmon
Total Cheats: 2.5 from the oil and the salmon

Dinner: Chicken with Peruvian Green Sauce (2.5);
Cauliflower Rice (.5); 450g of sautéed Spinach (you've earned a
cheat!); 125ml glass of wine (1)
Total Cheats: 4.5 (3.5 if you eat the spinach),

**Cheats: You've used six Cheats here. If you want the wine,
eat the greens after 5 p.m.**

Day 4
Breakfast: South of the Border Eggs or 2 scrambled eggs
Total Cheats: 0!

LUNCH: Butternut Squash Soup or Weight Loss Short cut Soup (1 Cheat); 1 serving of Easy Italian Baked Turkey (1.5 Cheats)
Total Cheats: 2 – from the oil or coconut milk and turkey

SNACK: Apple with 1 tablespoon of almond butter (1 Cheats)
Total Cheats: 1 – from the apple and almond butter

DINNER: Japanese Chilli Salmon (2 Cheats); Leftover Cheat-Free Stir-fry; cucumber or tomato salad (0); large cup of herbal tea
Total Cheats: 2.5 – from the salmon, oil, and avocado

Cheats: You've used five cheats. You have one remaining.

Day 5
BREAKFAST: Chocolate Raspberry Torte Shake
Total Cheats: 0 (first protein, fat is free!)

LUNCH: The Famous Puréed Energy Soup with Leftover Chilli Asian Salmon Stir-fry
Total Cheats: 3 – from the coconut milk, salmon, and oil

DINNER: Insane Man Hunger Chilli or Ginger Salmon with Bok Choy and Spinach; The Famous PEERtrainer Energy Soup

Cheats: You've had five cheats. You have one remaining cheat.

Day 6
BREAKFAST: Chocolate Almond Sea Salt Shake
Total Cheats: 0!

LUNCH: Slow Cooker Chicken and Spinach Soup; Sweet potato (2)

IF EATING OUT: Chipotle bowl (chicken, ½ serving of beans, lettuce, salsa, golf ball-size portion of avocado). If from home, 2 servings of soup with a serving of chicken. Or 2 pieces of salmon sashimi and a large mixed green salad with hot green tea
Total Cheats: 3

DINNER: Bacon Avocado Burgers (3 Cheats); 225g of broccoli; sautéed spinach; one piña colada (1 Cheat) or 125ml glass of wine
Total Cheats: 4 – you earned 1 Cheat from the greens! from the meat, bacon, avocado, coconut milk, and pineapple juice or wine

Cheats: You've used six Cheats. You have none left.

Day 7
BREAKFAST: Power Workout Breakfast or Carrot Cake Shake Or two hard-boiled eggs with leftover vegetables
Total Cheats: 0 Cheats!

LUNCH: Mediterranean Gourmet Power Bowl with optional extras (1 Cheat)
Total Cheats: 1 – from the oil and goat's cheese

DINNER: 100g grass-fed Steak or Orange Sauce over fish and Salad and ⅓ of avocado (2.5 Cheats) or Mint and Shallot Halibut with Kale and Oven-Roasted Tomatoes with greens
Total Cheats: 2.5 – from the steak or halibut, avocado, and oil

Cheats: You've had three and a half Cheats. You have two and a half left!

The Cheat Incentives

There is one more way you can earn two extra Cheats this week!

The Cheat Incentive for Week Three is:

You can earn **two extra cheats for the week** if you send yourself an email in the evening, every day this week, detailing everything you're appreciative of. The email should have the subject line of tomorrow's date and you should send it in the evening so you can read it the following morning.

List everything you're excited about or grateful for. It can be the smallest thing, like finding hairbands for a pound, to big important things like being thankful that your partner or parents are in good health. The list should include anything you're personally excited about – not everything on the list has to be profound or life-changing. I've literally included, "I'm so psyched about adding a third blanket to my bed because I'm finally warm at night!".

Week Three To Do

- ✦ Hurray! You're through the three weeks. Record your weight, review your goal and keep going.

Week Three Exercise Plan

- ✦ Complete Week Three of the Cheat Lifestyle Programme Fitness Plan.
- ✦ Aim to complete 30 minutes of continuous walking a day.
- ✦ Find your local pool and get in! Swimming is often overlooked, but is a great workout as whilst it can be high intensity there is very little impact on your joints. Start off small by completing 10 minutes of continuous swimming.

CHAPTER 8

·

Your Magic Fridge

How to Buy and Cook Smart

"It's impossible," said Pride. "It's risky," said Experience. "It's pointless," said Reason. "Give it a try," whispered the Heart.

I want to start this chapter by saying that reading this chapter is entirely optional. I've discovered that some people find "prepping" for a new way of eating helpful while others hate the process and just want to start the programme already!

The Magic Fridge is the biggest short cut there is to eat The Cheats and Eats Lifestyle Programme way. It will tell you not only what to get rid of from your refrigerator and cupboards but also what you should buy at the supermarket, from spices that help the Eats taste great to the Eats themselves so you reduce the chances of finding yourself staring into the fridge wondering what you're going to eat.

The Magic Fridge does not include recipes for low-fat cheesecake or wholewheat pizza. The reasons why should be obvious: first, we don't advocate for fake "healthy" foods on The Cheats and Eats Lifestyle Programme. We concentrate on meals made with whole, natural, actually healthy foods. The Magic Fridge focuses on the foods that should make up 80 per cent of your plate at every meal – the Eats that give you the high nutrients necessary for sustainable, and hunger-free weight loss.

I'll be honest. I would still rather pick up a slice of pizza any day of the week than cook a cheat-free meal. A slice of pizza is fast, tastes great and is really easy – but unfortunately, now that I'm over 40, I can't control my portions any more. One slice of pizza leaves me hungry and I end up gorging on almost the whole lot. The solution is creating high-nutrient meals that taste great, which don't require slaving in the kitchen all day – and that's what the Magic Fridge will give you.

For those of you who love food and love to cook, you're going to love what the Magic Fridge does for you – it's basically a sous chef in the form of a chapter. The fact is, if I had to choose between working all day in the kitchen to make a delicious meal or eating bland food, I wouldn't have been able to sustain my weight loss of over four stones. But with the Magic Fridge, you don't have to make that choice. It helps you create truly delicious, low-cheat, or even cheat-free meals without being in the kitchen all day.

Now, when I take the time to cook I know that it's an investment. What do I mean by saying it's an investment? Here's how I like to think of it: **If I spend time making food, it will be the gift that keeps on giving. I may spend 45 minutes making something that tastes great, but I'll see the results on the scale. And, if I make extra, I won't have to cook later today, tomorrow or later this week!**

I'll make a staple, such as grilled chicken, or the greens tapenade, which will last me for a few days in the fridge so I can grab it anytime I want to make a salad. If I make a soup, I'll make a lot of it so it lasts a few days or can be put in the freezer for later consumption.

When I first mentioned the concept of a constant resource of good, nutrient-rich food to my husband, he remarked that it reminded him of an Indonesian story he heard as a child, called The Magic Pot about a rice bowl that was always filled with food – and that's why I decided to name this chapter the Magic Fridge because that's what it's going to feel like: a fridge filled with food.

You can go to the supermarket and start this today. Think of it as a fun adventure where you're replacing the old with the new. There are four easy steps to the Magic Fridge:

1. Clean Out What's Not Working for You
2. Buy Essential Kitchen Tools
3. Fill Your Fridge with Must-Have Foods
4. Take Spice Short cuts

1. Clean Out What's Not Working for You

The number one thing I tell people interested in weight loss to do is to clean out their cupboards and their fridge. The rule of thumb is to clear out anything that you know is bad for you and takes five minutes or less to prepare and eat. When you're starving, you're going to turn to those foods if they are available in the cupboard or in the fridge for you to eat. By removing the foods you know are bad for you, you eliminate that option.

Willpower goes out the window when you're face-to-face with a bag of crisps. Be honest with yourself and get rid of anything that falls into the category of a food that's easy, tasty and is a Cheat. I already hear what you're thinking: "There's no way my husband/wife/boyfriend/girlfriend/son/daughter/kids/room-mate is going to let me do that. My husband used to regularly bring home a delicious cake from the store. I asked him not to – I couldn't resist them! – and he replied, you obviously don't know men and hunger. He refused to stop. (He also used to bring home tubs of ice cream but for some reason, that wasn't a problem for me. Ice cream just wasn't a trigger food, but that cake in the fridge was.) I knew that the moment I had a bad day, I was going straight to that cake. It took two years for him to listen but he finally did and stopped bringing home the cake. Don't give up asking for what you need. And after your room-mate/boyfriend/girlfriend/wife/husband/kids eat the delicious foods you prepare as part of your diet, they might be tempted to give up whatever food is tempting you and try The Cheats and Eats Lifestyle Programme way, too! You never know...

2. Buy Essential Kitchen Tools

The second step is to make your life easier by buying a few key kitchen tools. You may already have some of these in your kitchen! (Note that I assume that you already own a saucepan, a casserole dish, and other true basics.) There's no need to go "fancy" and buy luxury brands. Just shoot for something that has great reviews online or is a trusted brand, like OXO, Kenwood, Teflon and others.

The Five Essential Kitchen Tools

1. A Hand Blender

It's relatively inexpensive and is key to making healthy soups and purées. Don't try to use your existing food blender; it's not the same. The engine of a typical blender can be easily overwhelmed and burn out puréeing vegetables and greens. Using a hand blender makes it easy to make greens like spinach and kale taste delicious, by pulverising them and bringing out their nutrients. Once pulverised, you can mix the greens with whatever base or taste you want, like salsa or guacamole. Typically priced around fifteen pounds, a hand blender is a wise investment, especially if you like soups, sauces and shakes.

2. A Rice Cooker ... For So Much More Than Rice

You'll find that this is an incredible time-saving tool. You put your food in, walk away, and come back to it completely ready. Quinoa and vegetables can be made in a rice cooker incredibly fast and there's no need to even turn the stove on!

3. Freezer-Safe Containers

These are a lifesaver when you choose to cook in bulk. You can use them to freeze soups, stocks, sauces and traditional proteins. Buy a couple in a variety of sizes to try at first, and later you can buy more in the sizes you use most often, if needed.

4. A Great Knife and a Cutting Board

Ok, so technically these are two tools but they work hand-in-hand. Cutting vegetables will be much, much easier with a good knife than a substandard one. Buying a cutting board that is strong and durable will make a difference, too. If you don't like what you have now, this is a good excuse to buy replacements.

5. Two Large Salad Bowls

Many salad bowls are smaller than they should be, and that's because people think salads should be a side dish. On Cheat System, they are definitely not side dishes! Buying two large salad bowls will help you mix up a salad quickly and easily. And buying two makes it more likely that you'll have one clean when you want to make a salad! Make sure they're big enough to include not just greens but veggies, a protein and your dressing without making a mess.

Other handy kitchen tools can include a good slotted spoon, which is great for sautéing kale and other greens, a large stockpot, which allows you to make soups in bulk and store the rest directly in the fridge, and a water pitcher, which has been shown to increase the amount of water you'll drink during the day more than just relying on filling up your glass from the tap or using bottled water. Also, if you have a pitcher of water, it's super easy to flavour the entire pitcher with cucumber, lemons or limes, just like they do at the best spas.

3. Fill Your Fridge with Must-Have Foods

I want you to have at least two go-to foods in your fridge at all times. These are Eats that you love, which you can literally pull out and eat on the spot. Having these in your fridge is an insurance policy for when you feel like "you're so hungry you could eat a house." These should be healthy, energy-filled snacks and foods that are easy to prepare, that you don't have to think about too much to create a meal out of. Some of my favourites include hummus, cucumbers, tabbouleh, quinoa with mixed greens, avocado squeezed with lemon, and sliced tomato-and-cucumber salad, beans, sweet potatoes, chicken breasts, chilli, hard-boiled eggs, and soups. Soups are always at the top of my list. They are the ultimate Magic Fridge staple.

The list goes on and on and can be anything you want, provided your go-to foods are Eats. Having these on hand will help you make the right choices when you're starving and want food now.

There are three different kinds of foods that I want you to get used to having in the house and buying every single time you're in the supermarket.

The Three Must-Have Foods In Every Magic Fridge

1. Frozen vegetables

This can be whatever you like, but I want you to have some vegetables and better yet, some greens such as spinach and kale, that only take a few minutes in the microwave to prepare whenever you're hungry.

At all times, have at least two bags of frozen spinach or kale in your freezer. Organic is more expensive per bag but the nutrient content doesn't change from frozen to fresh, or organic to non-organic. Yes, buying organic is preferable but if that's too expensive for you, non-organic frozen greens are fine. Buy frozen vegetables and you'll always have something on hand to up the nutrient content of everything you eat.

2. Huge containers of fresh greens, spring greens and spinach

You can literally throw these into every meal you make on Cheat System, so every meal that you eat has more nutritional "heft." I like to have fresh, pre-washed salads and greens in my fridge because I'll add some to every meal I make. If you can do fresh, do fresh!

You can stick fresh spinach leaves in any smoothie you make because it's completely masked by the other flavours in the smoothie. (I do this when I make smoothies for my kids.) You can throw fresh spinach in rice, beans, wraps, dips, underneath a main dish like salmon or chicken, even in omelettes. It's really versatile and often, the flavour of spinach "disappears" when you have stronger flavours mixed in. Try it!

3. Condiments for the spice short cuts

Right now you probably have condiments such as ketchup, mayonnaise and soy sauce – which often have added ingredients and loads of sugar and fat. You can replace the flavours of those condiments with the ingredients for the spice short cuts we're going to share with you. But in terms of a shopping list for the condiments that make up the spice short cuts, you should buy and have on hand the following: garlic, fresh limes and lemons, mustard, chilli flakes, olive oil, cumin, turmeric, adobo or peri peri (spice blend), avocados, coriander, ginger, wasabi, oregano, basil, thyme and coconut milk. It's Ok if these are in dried form, though fresh is usually a little bit more flavourful. But do what you are able to do!

4. Take Spice Short cuts

One of the best ways to lose weight and love your food is to discover what flavours and spices you love. What is it that you love about the taste of pasta meat sauce? To replicate the flavour of a tasty Italian sausage sauce you can use tomatoes with basil, thyme, oregano, bay leaves and chilli flakes in a recipe for a healthy tomato soup that tastes like the sauce you love.

It's really easy to use spices to create delicious meals that taste similar to those bad-for-you "Cheat" foods. And once you start to use the spice short cuts listed here, you will develop a sense of what works together to make meals taste great. Feel free to experiment with your spice rack and your must-have condiments.

These spice combos make anything taste great!

+ **Fresh lime, coriander and chilli flakes** for Mexican-inspired meats, fish, soups and vegetables
+ **Lemon, olive oil and fresh garlic** for Mediterranean-style fish or salads
+ **Mustard, olive oil and lemon** for grilled vegetables, salads and chicken; you can give this a little kick by using a hotter mustard
+ **Coriander, avocado and lemon purée**, which adds a crisp flair to vegetables and salads
+ **Cumin, turmeric and ginger** for a Middle-Eastern, Indian-inspired mix to chicken, beans and meat
+ **Oregano, basil and thyme** for Italian-inspired meals and great for vegetables, chicken, and fish

- **Curry powder or garam masala** for Indian flavours
- **Ginger, garlic and red onion**, which is great for all meats (it's the base used for Chicken Tikka)
- **Wasabi, lemon and ginger** for Japanese-inspired fish and vegetables such as asparagus and broccoli
- **Coconut milk, chilli flakes, lime and onions** for Thai-inspired dishes and great for meats, vegetables and fish.

You can also use these spices to make easy salad dressings. The Magic Lime Dressing (page 182), which I think is quite delicious and incredibly versatile, only has three ingredients: the juice of two limes, a pinch of salt, and four shakes of chilli flakes. Though you can add ¼ of an avocado or some extra virgin olive oil to it, that's not necessary to make a delicious dressing for any salad.

Remember, the most important thing is that you learn what you like and you understand how not only to make great-tasting, nutrient-rich foods when you are at home cooking, but also how to find those same meals out and about in your day. If you find that you like tomatoes, onions and avocado, you will start to look for those combinations at restaurants and you will find them.

The Magic Fridge teaches you the basics of The Cheats and Eats Lifestyle Programme and it will create the good habits that will make you successful over the next three weeks. You'll start to see yourself eat better because it's easy to do when those foods are in your fridge; you'll feel more full because you're eating nutrient-rich foods; you'll take small steps to make vegetables taste better than you ever imagined and discover flavours that you never thought you'd like – and that you'll soon love.

PART THREE

Cheaters for Life

CHAPTER 9

The Cheating Gourmet

How to Create a Magic Kitchen (With 100 Recipes for Cheating and Eating!)

It's not the critic who counts...[it's] the man who is actually in the arena...

– Teddy Roosevelt

Almost a year ago, my mother-in-law – who is a brilliant, incredible chef – went to our local Indian store and bought over twenty-five common Indian spices to put in our cupboard. After she left, I put those spices away in a cupboard and I am not kidding when I say that I was afraid of that cupboard! For six months. I didn't know the first thing to do with cardamom, turmeric or black mustard seeds – and I really didn't want to. I knew there were lots of very healthy Indian dishes that my husband loved. But cooking seemed like so much time and effort even with spices I knew. Using spices I wasn't even remotely familiar with was way too intimidating for me.

Eventually, my mother-in-law came over again and showed me how to make her delicious fish curry. She took me through every single step and of course, since she was there, it turned out perfectly. But something else happened that day – I was no longer afraid of the cupboard. A few weeks later, once I had become confident in being able to make the curry, she showed me how to make another recipe. Now, a few years later, I know how to make three or four of my husband's favourite dishes – and trying a new Indian dish doesn't intimidate me anymore.

If you're the kind of person who gets nervous about using cookbooks and online recipes, or has no idea how your friends are able to make what they serve at dinner parties, you are not alone. If you are afraid to ask what the different herbs are in the produce section of your supermarket, you're not alone. Supermarkets can be incredibly overwhelming – I'm still intimidated by leeks; I actually don't even know what one would look like in a store! And even though a few friends of mine have explained how to prepare and cook leeks, I'm still nervous. I really love potato leek soup when I dine out, but will I ever make it for myself? Probably not – and that's Ok.

If you have no idea how to make hard-boiled eggs or prepare beans that aren't in a tin, you're definitely not alone. And if you're interested in learning, we're now going to teach you all those techniques. Everything you need to know to successfully Cheat and Eat – whether you want to cook, or want to avoid it like the plague – is in this chapter.

If you are at an advanced level – and love to spend time making new, healthy dishes – this chapter is for you, too. We've included advanced techniques and we teach you how to become a "cheating gourmet". Whatever your level, we have it here.

Your Magic Kitchen

I'm not going to assume you know anything about preparing or cooking food in this chapter. (So if you fancy yourself an amateur chef, you'll probably know a lot of the basics I'm going to share.) A lot of us – including myself – haven't spent days in our mum's kitchen or hours on the couch watching cookery shows learning how to make the perfect marinade or how to poach an egg. If you're that person, you're going to love the Magic Kitchen.

No One Is Perfect
You don't have to cook perfectly; in fact, most professional chefs would tell you that imperfect cooking typically ends up tastier than someone who follows a recipe or cookbook to the letter. If you don't have an ingredient, go without it. If you don't have the right pan, feel free to

use something similar. After all, an omelette that falls apart is just scrambled eggs: it has the same ingredients, the same taste, and the same number of Cheats. Don't beat yourself up over a scrambled egg. Don't make perfect the enemy of the good.

Cheatify, Cheatify, Cheatify!

The recipes in this chapter are designed for Cheating and Eating. However, if one of your favourite meals is not adapted in this chapter, you can always cheatify it. Think of Joel Fuhrman's term: G-BOMBS. Greens, Beans, Onions, Mushrooms, Berries, Seeds and Nuts. These are the best-bang-for-your-buck nutrients. Anytime you add onions, greens, cooked mushrooms, beans, vegetables, seeds, nuts, or berries to a recipe, you are successfully cheatifying that recipe. Think of the balancing scale: by adding those healthy Eats, you're tipping the whole meal in that direction. You'll notice we have cheatified a lot of common dishes in our recipes. For example, we cheatified burgers (Bacon Avocado Burgers, page 199), ranch dressing (Spicy Ranch Dressing, page 263), and even margaritas (Muscle Recovery Margaritas, page 276).

You can also do this when you're eating out. For example, recently our collaborator on this book went out to a Japanese ramen noodle restaurant. She ordered what seemed to be the healthiest option – the vegetable ramen soup, which had a vegetable broth, spinach noodles, chicken instead of pork, and lots of veggies – but the menu had an option to add kale and cabbage so she did that, asking for double portions of each. Instant cheatify!

The Basics

A lot of us have no idea how to cook rice, how to make greens taste great, or even what quinoa is. In this section, we'll go over a few basics that you might not find in the recipes themselves.

Cooking with (Less) Oil

A great way to use less oil when cooking is to let the pan properly heat first before adding it. Put the pan on the stove and let it heat up. After a few minutes, test the pan's temperature by taking a drop of water and flicking it to the pan. If the water sizzles and evaporates, your pan is hot enough. (If not, wait another minute and try again.)

This will not only allow you to use less oil, but will also prevent food from sticking to the pan. There's a lot less clean-up – and a lot fewer calories.

"Which Oil Should I Use?"

For most of our Cheat Lifestyle Programme recipes, we advocate using extra virgin olive oil or coconut oil. You might have heard that olive oil is toxic when heated – and while that is true, it only applies when you heat olive oil past its specific "smoke point".

Every oil has its own smoke point, which differs depending on how it's made and processed. As long as you don't heat the oil above that temperature, nothing bad will happen to you or your food. Here are the smoke points for the oils we recommend on this programme:

> Extra Virgin Olive Oil: 190°C/375°F
> Unrefined Coconut Oil: 175°C/350°F

Most of these oils won't approach their smoke points if you only heat your stove to medium (which is usually the case for most of our recipes). However, if you're going to cook something in the oven at high temperature – for example, if you are roasting vegetables or making sweet potato fries – you are better off using an oil with a high smoke point, such as coconut oil.

When buying oil to cook with you don't need to by the most expensive extra virgin olive oil. It's a waste when the flavour of the oil is lost in the dish. However, when you're making a recipe where the taste of the olive oil will really matter, adding some great or even flavoured extra virgin olive oil is ideal. Having garlic-infused extra virgin olive oil on hand to add to sautéed vegetables or to use in a salad dressing can add an extra dash of delicious.

How to Boil Eggs

Hard-boiled eggs are great to have on hand while Cheating and Eating. It's a quick protein when you're in a rush, is incredibly versatile (you can eat it on a salad, as part of a salad topping, or by itself), and can be a great alternative to hot eggs. Try adding smoked paprika, celery salt or even Tabasco sauce to hard-boiled eggs for extra flavour. Making hard-boiled eggs isn't difficult. First, put the eggs in a pot. Cover the eggs completely, with at least an inch of water over the entire egg(s). Bring the water to a boil. As soon as the water starts to boil, reduce the heat to low for 10–12 minutes so it's no longer boiling. Prepare another bowl with ice water. Remove the eggs with a slotted spoon and put them into the ice water carefully. Once the eggs are cooled, drain the water and store the eggs in a covered container in the refrigerator. Hard-boiled eggs last about five days in the refrigerator.

How to Make Greens Taste Great

Sautéed kale, spinach, Swiss chard, mustard greens – virtually any leafy green – can taste great. The trick is to prepare it correctly. To start, heat a frying pan or saucepan over medium to high heat. Add a little bit of oil, then add chopped greens. (If you like garlic, you can add minced garlic before you add in the greens.) Add 125ml of water, cover, and lower heat to medium.

After a few minutes, check on the greens to see if the water has evaporated; if it has, add a little more. Stir the greens around in the pan, so it cooks evenly. Depending on which green you're cooking and in what quantity, it will take 5–15 minutes to properly sauté your greens. If you're in doubt, taste them!

How to Make Quinoa

A lot of us are intimidated by quinoa. Perhaps it's because it's confusing to say (it's pronounced keen-wah) and when you look at it in its dry form, quinoa looks a lot like birdseed – which is no wonder because it is actually a seed. It's nutty and really satisfying. It's more nutritious and easier to make than traditional rice – and can be substituted for rice in nearly any recipe.

Typically 100g of dry quinoa makes 300g of cooked quinoa. You have to rinse quinoa first, to remove its saponins (a substance that naturally occurs on the outside of the quinoa grains to deter insects and birds). Rinse the quinoa by either using a fine sieve or by running fresh water over the quinoa in a pot and draining it.

Place 100g of quinoa and 200ml of water in a medium saucepan on medium-to-high heat and bring it to a boil. Once it's boiling, reduce the heat and simmer for 10–15 minutes, until all the water has evaporated. You'll be able to tell that the quinoa is done when its grains are translucent and its outer layer has separated.

How to Make Beans

Up until very recently, I was totally Ok using pre-made beans in tins. But once I learned how easy it was to make beans in bulk from scratch, I started doing that and rarely go back (though I do always keep tinned beans in my cupboard so I have some just in case). Beans you prepare yourself taste better than what comes in a can, and though it takes time I feel like making beans is totally worth it.

In order to cook beans from scratch, you need to soak beans first. (Lentils, split peas, and black-eyed peas don't need to be soaked.) Pick through the beans and discard any discoloured or shrivelled beans from the bag. Rinse the beans well and then put them in a large saucepan. If you are making a 450g bag , you will get about 1kg of cooked beans at the end. Cover the pan and refrigerate it overnight.

The next day, drain the soaked beans. Cover the beans with water and add any herbs or spices you want (avoid salt). Bring the beans and water to a boil, then simmer gently uncovered, stirring occasionally until the beans are tender. (The time depends on the type of bean you're making but it usually takes about 45 minutes to an hour.) Add more water if the beans are not completely covered at any point in the process. You can also toss beans in to a slow cooker – it's super easy and you don't have to watch at all! Beans can also be made in a pressure cooker and can save you loads of time.

When beans are tender, drain and use them as you want. If you're going to reserve some for later, immerse the beans in cold water until they are cool, then drain. You can freeze prepared beans into small serving portions by dividing between zip seal bags. This might sound like a lot of work, but I promise if you eat beans regularly, it's worth it!

Cheat Confetti

"Sprinkling" Cheats throughout your meals is the number one reason that readers find eating The Cheats and Eats Lifestyle Programme way to be so doable – and delicious. Throughout this chapter, you'll find a bunch of ideas that you can use for Cheat Confetti including

Parmesan crisps, bacon bits, power green confetti, cinnamon candied walnuts and toasted rosemary almonds! Use these ideas as a jumping off point to create your own your perfect Cheat Confetti. Maybe it will be adding candied walnuts to your salad, or adding bacon to anything.

Adding some Cheat Confetti – a topping to the party, not making it the main meal – is a great way to make a salad, a soup or a main meal taste delicious without going overboard or wasting a day's worth of Cheats. As a tip, don't have large amounts of Cheat Confetti in the fridge if you can't stay away from it. Only make individual servings if you think it's a potential trigger food.

The Recipes

In this chapter you will find **100 recipes** for cheating and eating. Some of these are our own creation and others have been kindly donated by readers and health experts that have contributed to this book.

Eat Any Recipe, Any Time

Though we separated our recipes into categories by what people typically eat, feel free to use any recipe for each of the three meals every day on The Cheats and Eats Lifestyle Programme. Personally, I love having Jackie's Vail Chophouse Salad (mine, adapted from the Vail Chophouse restaurant in the US, page 178) or the Savoury Rosemary Chicken Salad with Cheat Confetti Parmesan Crisps (pages 186 and 191) in the morning as breakfast, though I completely understand that most people have an image of what breakfast is in their head and a salad is not for breakfast. That's totally Ok.

When I lived abroad, I noticed that the locals ate things for breakfast like schnitzel or cucumber, tomato and onion salad, which was something I had never considered to eat at this time of day. Once I tried it, I realised why: these foods provided more energy than what I was used to eating for breakfast. And that's important because we do a lot after breakfast: we get ourselves ready for the day, get our families ready for the day and use our brain and body to do what we need to. There are no rules as to what you should eat at mealtimes and we often just get stuck in a rut. Try exploring new food ideas, breaking from the norm can make mealtimes more inspiring and even increase your nutrient intake and energy levels.

In many cultures, the biggest meal of the day is lunch and after eating that way for a while, it made sense to me. You've been going, going, going all morning; then you eat lunch and what do you do? You keep going, going, going.

Many people choose to eat a large dinner but maybe this isn't necessary given our lifestyle. After dinner we relax, we wind down (hopefully), we watch a little TV or read a book. We don't need a huge number of calories to *do* anything. We're not going, going, going at night the way we are during the day. Usually, we're going to go to bed in a few hours and rest.

So, if you can somehow trick your brain into eating dinner for breakfast, or even eating dinner for lunch, do it. If you can eat salmon and vegetables in the morning like people do in Japan (where people have been shown to live the longest and healthiest), do it.

But if you can't, you're in good company; a survey of our readers showed that 95 per cent feel the same way you do. Most people simply can't stomach the thought of eating dinner for breakfast. So, we've also included some traditional breakfast recipes, along with recipes for nutritious protein shakes. The shakes are a great meal, especially when you're pressed for time (which most of us are in the morning).

Count Your Cheats!

To help you out, we've also included the number of Cheats for each recipe. Keep in mind that the Cheats listed are for each individual serving. For example, the Insane Man Hunger Chilli recipe contains twelve servings. Each serving has two Cheats.

Counting By Serving…

Do keep in mind that the exceptions to the rule: first 100g of lean traditional protein or plant-based protein, the first tablespoon of a "good" fat for the day, the first fruit, the first cup of coffee are Eats and they are free but after you had a second helping of the fat or the protein it's a Cheat – remember Eats are unlimited, at any meal! So, for example, if you see a shake has one and a half cheats, remember it's free if it's your first meal of the day. These recipes have cheat numbers **without the exceptions to the rule figured in.**

If You Run Out of Recipes…
Try creating your own recipes based around the cheats and then filling up with the eats. You can also use the cheat sheet to work out how many cheats are in your favourite recipes or new ideas you would like to try from your favourite cookbooks or recipe websites.

Breakfast Recipes and Shakes

Shakes

Anti-inflammatory Shake

Servings: 1   **Cheats/Serving: 0**

Cheat free (after your first shake, it's 1.5)

1 scoop chocolate protein powder or unflavoured plant protein
    powder plus 1 tsp of cocoa
150g frozen blueberries
250g unsweetened almond milk
225g spinach

Add all the ingredients to a blender and blend until smooth.

Banana Chocolate Nut Shake

Servings: 1   **Cheats/Serving: 0**

Cheat free (after your first shake, it's 2)

1 banana, chopped
2 tsp almond butter
300ml unsweetened coconut milk
1 scoop chocolate protein powder or unflavoured plant protein
    powder plus 1 tsp of cocoa
6 ice cubes

In a blender, add the frozen banana, hemp seed, and coconut
milk. Blend until smooth. Add the protein powder and blend.
Add the ice cubes and blend until smooth.

Brian Rigby's Mint Chocolate Chip Cookie Smoothie

Servings: 1   Cheats/Serving: 0

Cheat free (after your first shake, it's 2)

The reason Brian uses oats in his shakes is two-fold: they're a great source of slow-digesting complex carbohydrates, which provide energy for hours, especially when combined with the protein and coconut milk in the shake; and they're naturally high in beta-glucan, a soluble fibre that promotes satiety, increases the health of our gut flora and lowers LDL (bad) cholesterol levels. The extra carbohydrates from the oats are key for active individuals to maintain good energy levels. The cacao nibs in this recipe are a great source of antioxidants.

250–500ml water
1 scoop chocolate protein powder or unflavoured plant protein powder plus 1 tsp of cocoa
250ml unsweetened coconut milk
1 dstsp of fibre, such as psyllium husks (add more if the texture allows)
1 tsp cacao nibs
1 packet loose leaf mint tea, run through a coffee grinder or mixed right into the shake
40g rolled oats

Add the ingredients into a blender, starting with 250ml of water. Blend, adding more water to achieve your desired thickness.

Carrot Cake Smoothie

Servings: 1   **Cheats/Serving: 0**

Cheat free (after your first shake, it's 1.5)

Thanks to Wendy Solganik, blogger of Healthy Girl's Kitchen, for this great carrot cake shake recipe.

1 scoop vanilla protein powder
250ml unsweetened coconut milk
120ml water
6 ice cubes
1 large carrot
½ tbsp chia seeds
1 tsp of fibre, such as psyllium husks
Pinch of cinnamon
Pinch of nutmeg
Pinch of ground cloves

Add all the ingredients to a blender and blend until smooth.

Chocolate Almond Sea Salt Shake

Servings: 1   **Cheats/Serving: 0**

Cheat free (after your first shake, it's 1.5)

Inspired by Chocolove!

4 ice cubes
1 scoop chocolate protein powder or unflavoured plant protein
with 1 tsp cocoa
250ml unsweetened coconut milk
1 handful frozen, blackberries
1 tsp vanilla extract
1 tsp fibre such as psyllium husks
Pinch of sea salt

In a blender, put the ice on the bottom and then add the other ingredients. Blend to desired consistency.

Chocolate Decadence Shake

Servings: 1   **Cheats/Serving: 0**

Cheat free (after your first shake, it's 1.5)

A quick note: the fibre can really thicken up the smoothie – some people like that and some don't. If you are new to extra fibre in your diet, you'll want to start small and work from there.

---

1 scoop chocolate protein powder or unflavoured plant protein
   powder plus 1tsp cocoa
250ml unsweetened coconut milk
6 ice cubes
1tsp fibre, such as psyllium husks
125ml water
100g greens (spinach, kale, whatever you have, fresh or frozen)
1 tsp cocoa powder
1 drop vanilla extract

In a blender, mix all the ingredients on a slow speed until the blended smooth. For those with a Vitamix, try and keep it smooth by slowing the speed to avoid foaming up the mix.

Chocolate Raspberry Torte Shake

Servings: 1   **Cheats/Serving: 0**

Cheat free (after your first shake, it's 1.5)

1 scoop chocolate protein powder
1tsp fibre, such as psyllium husks
250ml unsweetened coconut milk or almond milk
100g raspberries (frozen or fresh)
125ml water
6 ice cubes
6 nuts (optional)
Pinch of cinnamon to taste (optional)

Add all the ingredients in a blender and blend until smooth.

Mango Lassi Shake

Servings: 1   **Cheats/Serving: 0**

Cheat free (after your first shake, it's 2.5)

1 cup unsweetened almond milk or coconut milk
1 scoop vanilla protein powder
½ mango, chopped
6 ice cubes

Add all the ingredients to a blender and blend until smooth.

Orange Creamsicle Shake

Servings: 1   **Cheats/Serving: 0**

Cheat free (after your first shake, it's 1.5)

250ml unsweetened coconut milk
½ orange, peeled
6 ice cubes
1 scoop vanilla protein powder
1 tsp fibre, such as psyllium husks
1 tsp chia seeds
125ml water

Combine the coconut milk, orange and ice cubes in a blender and blend until smooth. While this is blending, add the protein powder.

Continue to run the blender while you add the fibre and chia seeds. Add water until your shake reaches the desired consistency.

Pumpkin Pie Smoothie

Servings: 1   **Cheats/Serving: 0**

Cheat free (after your first shake, it's 1.5)

Remember, be sure when picking a protein powder to use a minimum of 20g of protein with no additives or sugar. Pea and rice protein or pea and potato is our recommendation.

50g pumpkin flesh
1 scoop vanilla protein powder
½ tbsp flaxseed meal
250ml unsweetened coconut milk
1tsp fibre, such as psyllium husks
1 tsp pure vanilla extract
Pinch of nutmeg
Pinch of cinnamon
6 ice cubes

Place all ingredients into a blender and blend for 30 seconds, or until smooth.

Triple Berry Smoothie

Servings: 1   **Cheats/Serving: 0**

Cheat free (after your first shake, it's 1.5)

100g frozen blueberries, raspberries and/or blackberries
120ml water
300ml unsweetened coconut milk
1 scoop vanilla protein powder
1 tbsp chia seeds
1tsp fibre, such as psyllium husks

Place the berries, water, coconut milk, protein powder and chia seeds in a blender and blend until smooth. While continuing to blend, add the fibre supplement. Blend until smooth.

Vanilla Cinnamon Ginger Shake

Servings: 1   **Cheats/Serving: 0**

Cheat free (after your first shake, it's 1.5)

1 scoop protein powder
250ml unsweetened coconut milk
½ mango, skin and stone removed
½ tsp fresh ginger, minced
1 tsp vanilla extract
Pinch of cinnamon

Add all the ingredients to a blender and blend until smooth.

Egg-Based Breakfasts

Bacon and Egg Scramble Cakes

Servings: 4   **Cheats/Serving: 2**

These freeze well: try freezing leftovers in individual plastic bags to easily reheat them later.

1 tbsp extra virgin olive oil
4 pieces of back bacon, rind removed and chopped
2 shallots, chopped
4 omega-3 enriched eggs
1 small handful of flat-leaf parsley, chopped
Fresh berries for serving

Preheat the oven to 180°C/350°F/Gas Mark 4

Heat the oil in a frying pan over medium heat. Once the pan is hot, fry the bacon and shallots for four minutes. Meanwhile, whip the eggs in a bowl for at least 45 seconds. Add the cooked bacon, shallots and parsley to the eggs and mix with a fork. Pour the mixture into muffin tins, until they are nearly full. Bake for 20 minutes or until the eggs are set. Serve with berries.

Meg's Mexican Breakfast Frying pan

Servings: 2   **Cheats/Serving: 2**

This recipe pairs wonderfully with sautéed kale, spinach, broccoli or cabbage.

1 tbsp extra virgin olive oil
200g hash browns or chopped boiled new potatoes
4 eggs
800g–1.2kg tinned black beans, drained and rinsed
250g salsa (you can use as much as you want, really)
120g salsa verde (optional)

Have a small and a large saucepan (with a cover) on the stove. Heat the large saucepan on high until hot. Add the olive oil and hash browns. Cover for three minutes, flip the hash browns and cover again.

After the hash browns have been flipped, heat a small saucepan on medium. When the pan is hot, crack the eggs and cook. I like eggs over easy, but you can cook them any way you'd like.

When the hash browns have cooked another three minutes, mix so that whatever side is less done is on the pan side. Add the black beans. When the black beans have heated up, add the salsa and salsa verde. When the salsa has warmed, remove from the heat and put on a plate. Top with the cooked eggs.

Nearly Cheat-Free Huevos Rancheros with Spicy Garlic Kale

Servings: 2   **Cheats/Serving: 2.5**

2 tbsp extra virgin olive oil
2 garlic cloves, minced or pressed (add more if you love garlic)
400g kale
300ml water
200g tinned black beans, drained and rinsed
4 eggs
250g salsa
Adobo or peri peri seasoning to taste
Dried chilli flakes to taste
Sea salt and ground black pepper to taste

Heat olive oil in a saucepan or a frying pan over a medium heat. When the oil is warm but not hot, add the garlic. Once you can smell the garlic, add the kale and water and cover.

While the kale is cooking, heat the black beans in a small pan.

In a separate bowl, use a fork to scramble the eggs adding a shake of adobo. Heat a small pan over a medium-high heat and begin to cook the eggs. When the kale is done cooking, add dried chilli flakes, sea salt and ground black pepper.

Simply Divine Egg, Bacon and Goat's cheese Omelette

Servings: 2   **Cheats/Serving: 3**

To make this even faster in the morning, use leftover stir-fry vegetables from the night before!

2 tsp extra virgin olive oil
½ onion, thinly sliced
4 garlic cloves
16 mushrooms, sliced

1 large handful of spinach
Sea salt and ground black pepper to taste
4 eggs
Bacon and goat's cheese confetti

Heat a frying pan over medium heat. Once heated, add the oil. Add the onions and cook until they're light brown. Add the garlic and cook for about a minute. Add the mushrooms and sauté for four minutes, and then add the spinach and cook for another minute. Season with sea salt and ground black pepper. Remove the vegetables from the pan and set aside.

In a small bowl, stir the eggs until they're smooth. Add them to the same frying pan and cook until the eggs are almost cooked like a pancake. Add the vegetable mixture (or leftover stir-fry vegetables) and the confetti on top, and then fold over the eggs to create your omelette.

South of the Border Eggs

Servings: 2   Cheats/Serving: 2.5

4 hard-boiled eggs, chopped
½ avocado, chopped
Tomato and jalapeño dip or salsa to taste

Mix ingredients in a small bowl.

Power Breakfasts

Power Workout Breakfast

Servings: 2   Cheats/Serving: 1

> 1 tbsp extra virgin olive oil
> ½ onion, chopped
> 400g broccoli florets, chopped
> 2 tbsp crushed walnuts
> 6 handfuls fresh spinach leaves
> 1 tbsp oregano
> 150g cooked lentils
> 1 tsp sea salt
> 6 basil leaves, chopped

Heat a pan over medium-high heat and add the olive oil and onions. Sauté the onions until they're brown, and then add the broccoli. If the pan is a bit dry at this point, add two tablespoons of water. Cook for four minutes.

Add the walnuts and stir, cooking for two minutes. Add the spinach leaves, oregano, lentils and sea salt and heat through.

Adjust the sea salt or oregano if needed, and garnish with basil before serving.

Scott's Summer Breakfast Salad

Servings: varies, depending on   Cheats/Serving:
ingredients used   0 + 1/protein serving

Use as much or as little of each ingredient as you like! This salad is endlessly customisable – just have fun!

> Mixed greens
> Fresh spinach

1 handful rocket
Chopped strawberries
Blueberries
Raspberries
Any seasonal stone fruit, chopped (peaches, pears, nectarines)
Protein of choice
Fruit-flavoured balsamic vinaigrette (these are found mostly at
 specialty stores that carry different olive oils and vinegars.)
Cheat Confetti Toasted Rosemary Almonds or Cinnamon
 Candied Walnuts (page 268, optional)

Combine the ingredients in a medium-sized salad bowl. (You
need to add a protein so this isn't a salad-as-meal.) Top with
half a tablespoon of dressing and mix. Garnish with the almonds
or walnuts.

Lunch Recipes

Soups

Beef Stroganoff Soup

Servings: 4   **Cheats/serving: 4.5**

450g grass-fed minced beef or beef fillet (cut into 5mm
 thick slices)
1 tsp sea salt
1 tsp ground black pepper
1 small onion, chopped
250g white mushrooms, sliced thinly
250ml beef stock
100ml light coconut milk
200ml coconut cream
1 medium courgette, peeled into noodles using a julienne peeler
1 large carrot, peeled into noodles using a julienne peeler

2 large garlic cloves, minced
1 tbsp Dijon mustard
Chopped fresh flat-leaf parsley or dill for garnishment (optional)

Lightly season the beef with sea salt and ground black pepper. In a saucepan over a medium-high heat, brown the beef and onion until the meat is browned and the onions are tender. Add the remaining ingredients except parsley or dill.

Bring to boil, then reduce the heat to low, cover and simmer for about 10 minutes

Uncover and simmer for about 10–15 minutes until the courgette and carrots are to the desired tenderness

Serve hot in bowls and garnish with parsley or dill, if desired.

Big Barley Soup

Servings: 4   **Cheats/Serving: 1.5**

1.5–2l low-sodium beef broth or home-made stock
1 large onion, chopped
2 medium carrots, chopped
2 celery stalks, chopped
1 green pepper, halved, deseeded and chopped
150g frozen peas
125g barley
½ tsp soy sauce or tamari
1 tbsp fresh basil, chopped or 1 tsp dried basil
Sea salt and ground black pepper to taste

Add all the ingredients to a slow cooker. Cook on a heat for 3–4 hours.

Chicken Piccata Soup

Servings: 8 **Cheats/ serving: 2**

250ml low-sodium chicken broth
2 lemons, juiced
4 skinless, boneless chicken breasts
3 tbsp olive oil
1 onion, finely chopped
3 cloves of garlic, finely chopped
150g artichoke hearts, drained and chopped
3 tbsp capers (optional)
1 tsp freshly ground black pepper
1 tbsp flat-leaf parsley, chopped

In a zip seal bag, combine the broth, lemon juice and chicken. Marinate overnight.

The next day, in a medium frying pan, heat the oil over medium heat, sauté the onion and garlic until softened, about two minutes.

Remove the chicken from bag (reserving the marinade) and place in frying pan to brown on each side, 5–10 minutes. Add the artichoke hearts, capers, ground black pepper and reserved marinade.

Reduce the heat and simmer until the chicken is thoroughly cooked, about 10 minutes

Serve and garnish with parsley.

Chilled Summer Gazpacho

Servings: 4   **Cheats/Serving: 1**

Though you can eat this about a half hour after you make it, this chilled soup is best if you let it sit in the fridge for a day so the flavours can blend together. It's the perfect summer soup.

Feel free to experiment with different vegetables as well! All you technically need to make gazpacho is tomato juice, onion and coriander. Everything else is up to you!

1 red pepper
1 yellow pepper
1 orange pepper
1 green pepper
2 cucumbers, peeled
2 red onions, chopped
800g tinned chopped tomatoes
2 garlic cloves, minced
1–2 bottles of V8 vegetable juice (you can use tomato juice as
    well, though V8 is a better base)
Cayenne pepper to taste
Chipotle style hot sauce
Sea salt and coarsely ground black pepper to taste
Adobo or peri peri seasoning to taste
1 handful of coriander, chopped
1 handful of flat-leaf parsley, chopped
1 avocado, halved, de-stoned and sliced

Dice the bell peppers, cucumbers and onions to whatever size you'd like. Put bell peppers, cucumbers, onions, diced tomatoes, and garlic in a large stockpot that fits in your fridge. Add the V8 juice until the consistency of the soup is what you want. Mix well. Add the jalapeño, ground black pepper and seasonings. This soup's taste varies a lot based on the seasonings you use, so feel free to experiment until you get the taste you want.

Once the taste is right, Add the coriander and parsley and let the soup sit in your fridge for at least a half hour; or best of all, let it sit overnight. When ready to serve, add slices of avocado to the top. Yum!

My Mom's Chilli

Servings: 8   **Cheats/Serving: 1**

This chilli recipe is an easy one to double or triple if you have guests.

1 tbsp extra virgin olive oil
450g grass-fed minced beef or minced turkey
2 tomatoes, diced
400g tinned pinto beans, drained and rinsed
400g tinned kidney beans, drained and rinsed
1 onion, chopped
1½ tsp chilli powder
1 tsp sea salt
2 garlic cloves, minced
½ tsp ground cumin
250ml water

In a frying pan over medium heat, heat the oil. Add the meat and cook until it is browned.

Transfer beef and the remaining ingredients to a slow cooker, mix and cook for 2–3 hours and then turn the heat down to low until you're ready to serve.

Philly Cheesesteak Soup

Servings: 4   **Cheats/Serving: 3**

1 onion, chopped
100g mushrooms (optional)
1 green pepper, chopped
450g grass-fed stewing beef, cut into thin strips
¼ tsp fresh ginger, minced
¼ tsp chilli flakes
150g Parmesan cheese

Sauté the onion and mushroom in frying pan over medium-high heat for about 2–3 minutes. After the onion has softened, add the green pepper. Then add the meat, ginger and chilli flakes to the frying pan.

Cover and cook until the meat is to your preferred tenderness. Top with Parmesan cheese until melted. Remove from heat, then serve and enjoy!

Salads and Dressings

Avocado and Bacon Chicken Salad

Servings: 4   **Cheats/Serving: 2 + 1 cheat confetti**
                               serving of bacon

450g grilled chicken breast (pre-cooked, store-bought chicken
works here)
1 avocado
1 lemon
Sea salt and ground black pepper to taste
Cayenne pepper to taste
Cheat Confetti Bacon for garnish (page 190)

Cut the chicken and avocado into small chunks and place
in a bowl. Add the juice from the lemon and stir. Add the sea
salt, ground black pepper and cayenne pepper. Top with Cheat
Confetti Bacon and serve.

Boulder Athletic Recovery Salad/Asian Fusion Salad

Servings: 4   **Cheats/Serving: 2**

The bok choy in this recipe is super crunchy and makes an
excellent base that can support a variety of flavours. As you
develop the habit of adding bok choy to your salads, you'll find
yourself eating a lot of it. And, one head of bok choy has around
900mg of calcium! You can also add chopped spinach to this salad
for more nutrients.

450g boneless, skinless chicken thighs
1 head bok choy
1 bunch spring onions
Dressing
1 tbsp toasted sesame oil
Juice of 1 lemon (or more to taste)

1 tbsp honey (this is a must for the recipe)
1 tsp sea salt
Ground black pepper to taste
2.5cm piece of ginger
Crushed chilli flakes to taste
1 jalapeño or green chilli, finely chopped (optional)
Small handful of coriander, chopped
Almonds or almond butter

Heat a pan over medium heat. Once hot, add the chicken and cook through. Be sure to cut one piece of chicken open to ensure its cooked throughout (it's no longer dark pink). Once cooked, drain the fat, cool and chop. You can use all the chicken, or save half in the fridge to use later in a second batch. For a vegan option, substitute the chicken with tofu or similar.

Chop the bok choy and finely chop the spring onion. Toss them into a large bowl with the cooled chicken.

Using a food processor or blender, blend the dressing ingredients. You can really work the flavour here, and adjust to your own tastes.

Toss the dressing into the chicken mixture. If you want a spicier salad, add more spices. If you want a nuttier flavour, add more sesame oil. Top with parsley or coriander and almonds.

Tip: If you don't have almonds, use a tablespoon of almond nut butter.

Chaat Masala and Lime Dressing (cheat free!)

Servings: 2   **Cheats/Serving: 0**

Courtesy of Uma Naidoo, M.D.

Uma is a wonderful friend of ours who is a culinary delight. I highly encourage you to make her dressings! You can purchase chaat masala online or in specialist food shops.

2 tbsp chaat masala
1 lime, juiced
½ orange, juiced
1 tbsp white wine vinegar
Sea salt to taste
Lime zest to taste

Whisk ingredients together and store in an airtight container.

Caesar Dressing

Servings: 2   **Cheats/Serving: 0.5**

Sometimes you just want the taste of Caesar dressing but we all know it can make a large classic Caesar salad with croutons ordered at a restaurant more than 20 Cheats! Here is our version – and for those of you who are gluten free, we've made this for you.

2 fresh anchovies
3 garlic cloves
5 heaping tbsp low-fat Greek yogurt
3 tbsp tamari or light soy sauce
Juice of 1 lemon
1 tbsp Parmesan cheese
½ tsp sea salt
Freshly ground black pepper

Roughly chop the anchovies and garlic. Add all the ingredients to a blender or food processor and blend until smooth.

Serve with romaine lettuce and grilled chicken.

Creamy Chicken Salad

Servings: 4   **Cheats/Serving: 1.5**

450g grilled chicken breast
4 tbsp low-fat Greek yogurt
2 garlic cloves, minced
2 tbsp tamari or light soy sauce
Juice of ½ lemon
Sea salt and ground black pepper to taste

Cut the chicken breast into 1cm chunks and set aside.

Add the yogurt, garlic, tamari, lemon juice, sea salt and ground black pepper to a blender or food processor and blend until smooth.

Pour the dressing over the chicken and mix thoroughly.

Diced Chicken, Grape and Pecan Salad

Servings: 5   **Cheats/Serving: 2.5**

2 tsp apple cider vinegar or lemon juice
120g light or home-made mayonnaise
10 white, seedless grapes, halved
490g boneless, skinless, free-range chicken breasts, diced
3 sticks of celery, diced
30g pecans, chopped, or flaked almonds

In a pot, bring enough water to cover the chicken to a boil. Once it's boiling, add the chicken and cook for 15–20 minutes, or until the chicken is no longer pink in the centre. Remove the chicken from the water and let it cool. Once it's cool enough to handle, shred the meat.

In a large mixing bowl, combine all the ingredients and mix well. Serve chilled.

Green Tea, Poppy Seed and Mint Vinaigrette

Servings: 4   **Cheats/Serving: 0.5**

Courtesy of Uma Naidoo, M.D

125ml chilled green tea
60ml fresh squeezed orange juice with pulp (for texture)
2 tbsp extra-virgin olive oil
1 tbsp fresh mint
1 tbsp poppy seeds
⅛ tsp ground ginger powder
Sea salt to taste
Orange zest to taste

Shake ingredients together and store in an airtight container.

Jackie's Vail Chophouse Salad

Servings: 2   **Cheats/Serving: 2**
                                    (Chicken), 3 with optional bacon

There is no extra dressing in this recipe. The avocado and lemon, along with the sea salt and ground black pepper, give this salad the perfect moist consistency.

200g skinless, boneless salmon fillets
Juice of 1 lemon or 1 lime
Sea salt and ground black pepper to taste

or

200g lean chicken breast
1 tsp olive oil
Sea salt and ground black pepper to taste

225g mixed greens
¼ red onion, thinly sliced into half moons
½ avocado
Juice of ½ lemon (optional)
Sea salt and ground black pepper to taste (optional)
5 cashews, chopped or 1½ bacon slices, crumbed (optional)

To Make the Salmon:

Preheat the oven to 200°C/400°F/Gas Mark 6.

In a baking dish, place a sheet of parchment paper large enough to wrap the salmon. Place the salmon on the parchment paper. Add lemon juice, sea salt, and ground black pepper on top. Seal the parchment paper around the salmon. Bake for 22 minutes, checking the fish after 15 minutes. It's done when it is easily flaked with a fork.

To Make the Chicken:

Place a saucepan over medium heat. Add the olive oil.

Slice the chicken into pieces. Season and cook for four minutes each side until the chicken is no longer pink when cut open.

To Assemble the Salad:

In very large mixing bowl, add the greens, onion, avocado, lemon juice, sea salt, ground black pepper and cashews or bacon, if desired. Mix well. Add the warm salmon or chicken and mix.

Apple, Grapefruit and Coriander Salad

Servings: 2   **Cheats/Serving: 0**

You can substitute two mangoes for the grapefruit in this recipe.

---

1 large apple, peeled and cut into 5cm long strips
2 small red onion, thinly sliced into rings
2 red grapefruits, peeled and segmented with membranes
*   removed*
Juice of 1 lime
2 tbsp coriander, chopped
Sea salt to taste
Cayenne pepper to taste

In a large bowl, gently mix all the ingredients. Chill before serving.

Julie's Taco Salad

Servings: 6   Cheats/Serving: 3

Julie was a college room-mate of mine and she is obsessed with perfecting the Taco Salad. This is her best!

450g ground turkey meat
1 pack of taco seasoning
120ml tomato passata
Worcester sauce (to taste)
400g tinned kidney beans, drained and rinsed
1 head of lettuce, chopped or torn into small pieces
1 tomato, chopped
200g grated cheddar cheese
Tortilla chips, crushed
1 jar of salsa (optional)

Brown the turkey in a frying pan over medium heat. Drain the meat, put it back into the frying pan and add the taco seasoning, passata and Worcester sauce. Stir well. Add the kidney beans and then set the mixture aside.

Prepare the salad by layering the lettuce, meat, and kidney bean mixture in a bowl. Add the tomato and cheese. Mix. Now add the desired amount of crushed tortilla chips on top. Serve with salsa on the side to add as dressing, if desired.

Lemon Almond Miso Sauce

Servings: 8   **Cheats/Serving: 0.5**

This sauce is wonderful with any protein, or even as a dressing on mixed greens.

4 heaped tbsp almond butter
2 heaped tbsp sweet white miso
800ml water, for thinning
1 lemon

In a saucepan over a medium heat, add the almond butter, miso, water, and lemon zest. Whisk until integrated, 5–10 minutes. Add the lemon juice and mix.

Lemon Wasabi Dressing

Servings: 1   **Cheats/Serving: 0**

This dressing is wonderful on fish.

Juice of 2 lemons
1 tsp wasabi
1 tsp tamari or light soy sauce

Mix together all the ingredients, and then serve.

Magic Lime Dressing

Servings: 1   Cheats/Serving: 0

Juice of 2 limes
Sea salt to taste
4 shakes of chilli flakes

Add ingredients to a small bowl and mix well.

The Mediterranean Espagna Salad

Servings: 2   Cheats/Serving: 2

The "Med" is one of my favourite restaurants in Boulder and this happens to be one of their best salads!

Field greens
½ cucumber, chopped
12 baby plum tomatoes (halved)
8 strawberries, sliced
2 tbsp toasted pine nuts
½ red onion, finely chopped
Magic Lime Dressing (see above)
Protein of choice
50g goat's cheese

Toss the greens, cucumber, tomatoes, strawberries, pine nuts, and red onion in a bowl. Add the dressing and toss well to coat. Top the salad with your favourite protein and goat's cheese.

Mexican City Chicken Salad

Servings: 4   **Cheats/Serving: 1.5**

450g grilled chicken breast
250g Pico de Gallo (recipe below)
200g tinned black beans, drained and rinsed (optional)
Pico De Gallo
1 tomato
¼ red onion
¼ jalapeño or green chilli pepper
¼ avocado
2 tbsp coriander
Juice of ½ lime

Cut the chicken breast into small chunks and place in a medium-sized bowl.

To make the Pico de Gallo, finely dice the tomato, onion and jalapeño. Dice the avocado and chop the coriander before adding to the bowl. Squeeze the lime juice over the tomato mixture and then mix well.

Mix in the chicken and beans and serve.

Mung Dal Salad

Servings: 2   Cheats/Serving: 0

Substitute other sprouted beans for mung beans if you wish.

200g split yellow mung beans
1 tomato, chopped
1 cucumber, peeled and chopped
3–4 red radishes, chopped
½ red onion or 3–4 spring onions, chopped
2 tbsp fresh ginger, minced
½ jalapeño or green chilli finely chopped
3 tbsp lemon juice
1 small handful of coriander, chopped
Sea salt to taste

Rinse the beans in water. Add the beans to a small saucepan and cover with fresh water. Bring to the boil and simmer for 15 minutes until tender then drain and leave to cool.

Place the beans in a mixing bowl with the remaining ingredients and mix thoroughly.

Night Eater's Best Friend Salad

Servings: 3   Cheats/Serving: 1

This salad is designed for eating between 4 and 6 p.m. It contains a load of micronutrients. Ideally, you'll eat the bulk of this yourself, but share if you must. In our experience, it is impossible to make too much salad. If you have someone in your home who is not a salad eater, this is a great way to convert them to the power of a massive salad.

This salad is delicious, so it helps you realise that eating high volumes of greens can be done easily. As our friend Dr. Joel

Fuhrman says, the salad is the main course. This one is awesome if you like a crunchy, flavourful eating experience.

---

3 hearts of romaine lettuce
2 handfuls salad mix
½ an avocado
Juice of 1 lemon
1 tsp Dijon Mustard
2 garlic cloves, crushed and diced
1 tbsp extra virgin olive oil
Sea salt and ground black pepper to taste
Cheat Confetti of your choice

Chop the three romaine hearts into 2cm strips and place in a large bowl. Add your salad mix of choice. Dice the avocado and add it to the bowl. In a small bowl, whisk together the remaining ingredients (except for the Cheat Confetti) until emulsified.

Mix the dressing from the small bowl into your salad greens, and then top with your Cheat Confetti.

Pear and Roquefort Salad

Servings: 4   **Cheats/Serving: 1**

1 red William or comice pear
1 conference pear
½ red onion, sliced
1 tbsp Roquefort cheese
1 handful walnuts
Freshly chopped parsley to taste
Dressing
Juice of 1 lemon
1 drop good mustard
1 squeeze of honey
½ tbsp extra virgin olive oil

Wash the fruit, and then slice the pears and place them on a plate, alternating colours. Add onion slices. Top with the cheese, walnuts and parsley.

In a small bowl, add the dressing ingredients and whisk until it thickens. Pour over the pears.

Savoury Rosemary Chicken Salad

Servings: 4   **Cheats/Serving: 2**

If you're buying the chicken fresh from the counter or butcher, ask them to cut it into squares or strips for you. Just mention you're making a stir-fry or salad and they'll be happy to do it. This saves lots of time for you when you're preparing this dish.

700g mixed greens
1 tbsp freeze-dried dill or 1 fresh dill sprig
3 tbsp fresh coriander (optional)
3 tbsp Italian parsley
½ tbsp extra virgin olive oil
450g lean chicken breast
2 tbsp fresh rosemary, chopped
½ red onion, finely sliced
½ avocado
Sea salt and ground black pepper to taste
Juice of ½ lemon or 2 tbsp apple cider vinegar

In a large salad bowl, mix the greens, dill, coriander, and parsley.

In a saucepan over medium heat, add the olive oil and then the chicken. Add the rosemary, spreading it evenly over the chicken. Cook for 8–10 minutes, flipping three or four times during the cooking. Be sure to cut a piece of chicken open to make sure it's cooked throughout (no longer dark pink). Set the chicken aside.

Add the onions, avocado, chicken, sea salt and ground black pepper to the mixed greens. Add the lemon juice and mix well.

Simple French Dijon Dressing

Servings: 2   **Cheats/Serving: 1**

1 tbsp of Dijon mustard (no honey, no spice, straight Dijon)
Juice of 2 lemons
2 garlic cloves, chopped
2 tbsp extra virgin olive oil
Pinch of sea salt

Blend all the ingredients together.

Tequila-Pineapple Dressing

Servings: 2   **Cheats/Serving: 0.5**

Courtesy of Uma Naidoo, M.D.

For a non-alcoholic version of this dressing, substitute apple cider vinegar for the tequila. This will also lower the calorie count.

25ml tequila
60ml lime juice
100ml sparkling water
25ml lemon juice
100g fresh pineapple purée
Sea salt to taste

Combine ingredients and store in an airtight container.

Tex-Mex Salad with Crisps

Servings: 2   **Cheats/Serving: 2.5**

This is my favourite salad, even after years of eating it! The best part is the Tex-Mex Tabbouleh. In addition to using it for this salad, I use it for lots of other recipes since it's delicious and completely cheat-free (if you leave out the crisps).

If you don't have the ingredients for the Tex-Mex Tabbouleh, just combine salsa or Pico de Gallo with cooked quinoa.

8 huge handfuls mixed greens, chopped
½ head cabbage, chopped
200g tinned chickpeas, drained and rinsed (optional)
200g Tex-Mex Tabbouleh (recipe opposite and this is equal to half the recipe)
½ avocado
Juice of 2 limes

Sea salt to taste
Chilli flakes to taste
1 gigantic handful plain sea salt crisps (optional)

Place the mixed greens and cabbage in a bowl. Add the chickpeas, Tex-Mex Tabbouleh, avocado, juice of 2 limes, sea salt and chilli flakes. Crumble the crisps on top, if desired, and toss well.

Tex-Mex Tabbouleh

360g cooked quinoa
1 tomato, chopped
1 cucumber, halved and seeds removed, and then chopped
½ red onion or 2 spring onions, chopped
½ jalapeño or green chilli, chopped (optional)
Juice of ½ lime
2 tbsp coriander
Sea salt to taste

Mix together the quinoa, tomato, cucumber, red onions and jalapeño. Add the lime juice and coriander and mix well. Add sea salt to taste.

Watermelon, Mint and Caper Dressing (cheat free!)

Servings: 4   Cheats/Serving: 0

Courtesy of Uma Naidoo, M.D

½ cup watermelon juice (blend seedless watermelon to make
  fresh juice)
½ cup sparkling water
2 tbsp capers, puréed
1 tbsp mint, chopped
Sea salt to taste
Pinch of black pepper

Combine the ingredients and store in an airtight container.

Cheat Confetti for Lunch

Cheat Confetti Bacon

Servings: 4   Cheats/Serving: 1

Try to find an uncured bacon for this recipe.

4 streaky bacon rashers, sliced in half

Place a large frying pan over medium heat. Take the half-strips of bacon and place in the frying pan (no oil required). Every few minutes, flip until the strips are a crispy, golden brown. Be sure not to burn the bacon! You must be in the kitchen when you're cooking these.

Once crisp, remove from the pan and place on doubled paper towels. Blot any extra grease. Crumble each strip into small pieces and place into a small, airtight container. Serve atop your favourite salad or dish as Cheat Confetti.

Cheat Confetti Parmesan Crisps

Servings: 4   **Cheats/Serving: 0.5**

Use these as confetti atop salads, chicken or your favourite casserole. Double this recipe if you'd like to keep extra for your magic fridge.

10 tbsp finely grated Parmesan cheese

Place a small saucepan over a medium heat. When it's hot, spread grated Parmesan as evenly as possible in the pan. Do not stir or flip. When the Parmesan is light brown and an almost solid sheet, remove it with a fish slice. Allow it to cool, and then break it up into pieces.

Power Green Confetti

Servings: 4   **Cheats/Serving: 0**

This cheat-free confetti adds greens to any dish without compromising the taste. Serve with salad, soup or any favourite dish for colour or as "herbs".

225g greens (kale, spinach, whatever you like)
Favourite herbs (optional)

Put your washed greens and any herbs you'd like into a food processor. Process until they're finely chopped.

Protein Based and More:

The Base salad

Servings: 4   **Cheats/Serving: 2.5**

The perfect answer to your bacon lettuce and tomato sandwich, cheatified.

3 cooked bacon rashers
450g cooked salmon
1 tomato, sliced
Rocket or mixed greens
Very large romaine hearts
Pico de Gallo (page 183)

Layer the bacon, salmon, tomato, and rocket on a large romaine hearts or large cabbage leaves. Add the Pico de Gallo.

Chipotle Shrimp Fajitas with Avocado and Salsa

Servings: 4   **Cheats/Serving: 1.5 with the optionals**

1 tbsp extra virgin olive oil
450g raw king prawns
Chipotle sauce to taste
Chilli flakes to taste
2 red onions, finely sliced
1 green pepper, sliced
1 red pepper, sliced
80g button mushrooms, sliced (optional)
½ jalapeño or green chilli, finely chopped
Adobo or peri peri seasoning to taste
Round lettuce
Salsa (optional)
Avocado, diced (optional)
Black beans (optional)

Heat a frying pan over medium heat. Add the olive oil. Coat the shrimp in chipotle seasoning and place in the hot pan. After 1–2 minutes, add the chilli flakes, onions, peppers, mushrooms and jalapeños.

When the shrimp is no longer translucent and the vegetables have softened, add the adobo seasoning and heat through.

Create wraps with the round lettuce leaves, shrimp mixture, and salsa, avocado, or black beans.

Classic Italian Grilled Cheese

Servings: 2   **Cheats/Serving: 4**

1 tbsp extra virgin olive oil
4 slices of your favourite bread
3 slices of cheddar cheese
2 tsp dried Italian seasoning or dried oregano

Place a frying pan over medium heat. Add the olive oil to the pan. Prepare the sandwich by placing the cheese and herbs on one slice of bread, then placing the other slice of bread on top.

Cook the sandwich in the frying pan until the bread is toasted and the cheese is melted, flipping the sandwich over at least once to toast both slices of bread.

Easy Foil Rosemary Chicken

Servings: 2   **Cheats/Serving: 1**

1 chicken breast
4 fresh rosemary sprigs
Sea salt and ground black pepper to taste

Preheat the oven to 180°C/350°F/Gas Mark 4.

Take two sprigs of rosemary and pull the leaves off the stem. Chop in quarters if possible (halves are Ok, too).

Place a piece of foil that will cover the chicken in a baking dish; place half of the rosemary underneath the chicken breast and then sprinkle the top with sea salt and ground black pepper. Add the remaining half of the rosemary to the top of the chicken and seal the foil.

Bake for 30 minutes.

Easy Italian Herb Baked Turkey

Servings: 4   **Cheats/Serving: 1**

450g boneless turkey breast
1 tbsp extra virgin olive oil
1 lemon or 1 lime
1 handful fresh herbs (basil and oregano)
1 tsp salt

Preheat the oven to 180°C/350°F/Gas Mark 4.

Set aside a piece of foil large enough to completely wrap the turkey breast.

Rub the turkey breast with oil. Place it on one side of the foil. Slice the lemon or lime and lay the slices on top of the turkey breast. Place the fresh herbs on top of the lemon or lime.

Fold the foil and roll the edges like a Cornish pasty. Bake on a baking tray or oven dish for 25–35 minutes.

Aubergine, Tomato and Mozzarella Italian Casserole

Servings: 4   **Cheats/Serving: 1 cheat per serving**

1 large aubergine
1 large, red tomato
100g fresh mozzarella
600g jar of tomato sauce (flavour of your choice but plain basil
  works well)
Fresh basil to taste

Preheat the oven to 180°C/350°F/Gas Mark 4.

Peel the aubergine, and then slice it into thin rounds. Slice the tomato and mozzarella into rounds.

In a baking dish, cover the bottom with the tomato sauce. Layer one slice of aubergine, one slice of tomato and one slice of mozzarella and place it in the dish, being careful to keep each tower separate. When you've finished your towers, top them with the fresh basil and a little more sauce. Bake for 35 minutes.

Fresh Spring Green Beans with Flaked Almonds

Servings: 2   **Cheats/Serving: 1**

450g fresh green beans, trimmed
½ tsp sea salt
1 tsp coconut oil
2 spring onions, chopped
30g toasted flaked almonds

Bring 4cm of water to a boil in a medium pot fitted with a steamer basket.

Sprinkle green beans with ¼ tsp sea salt and place in the steamer basket. Cover and steam for 10 minutes, or until the green beans are tender-crisp. Immediately plunge the green beans into an ice water bath to stop the cooking, and then drain them. Meanwhile, heat a non-stick frying pan over a medium-high heat. Add the oil once the pan is hot. Add the green onions and sauté for 2–3 minutes, or until they're soft. Add the green beans, nuts, and remaining sea salt, stirring until thoroughly heated.

Hot and Spicy Black Beans and Rice

Servings: 4   **Cheats/Serving: 0**

1 tbsp extra virgin olive oil
1 small onion, chopped
½ green pepper, chopped
200g tomatoes, diced
400g tinned black beans (drained but reserve the liquid)
½ tsp thyme
1 tsp garlic, minced
3 tbsp apple cider vinegar
½ tsp hot sauce
300g cooked white or black rice

In a frying pan over a medium heat, heat the olive oil. Once the oil is hot, cook the onion and green pepper until they are tender. Stir in the tomatoes, drained beans, thyme and garlic. Cook for three minutes.

Add the vinegar, hot sauce, and reserved bean liquid. Cook for five more minutes. Serve over rice. Enjoy!

Mediterranean Gourmet Power Bowl

Servings: 4   **Cheats/Serving: 0.5 (1 with "Optionals")**

Mediterranean cuisine is one of my favourites. It feels so fresh and clean and tastes like spring. In this recipe, if you'd like to be extra fancy, you can roast eight garlic cloves at 200°C/400°F/ Gas Mark 6 for 25 minutes instead of using the three cloves of chopped garlic.

250g uncooked quinoa
400g artichoke hearts, drained
15 sun-dried tomatoes, quartered
Spinach, kale or bok choy finely chopped in a food processor
  (enough to help reach a daily goal of 225g greens) (optional)
2 tbsp extra-virgin olive oil
3 garlic cloves, chopped
Small handful of fresh basil
3 shakes crushed chilli flakes (or more to taste)
Sea salt to taste
30g goat's cheese, crumbled (optional)

Prepare the quinoa according to the packet directions. It's usually 1 part quinoa to 2 parts water. I highly recommend preparing it in a rice cooker. If you don't have a rice cooker, just bring the water to a boil, add the quinoa, reduce the heat, cover and simmer for 15–17 minutes until it is fluffy.

While quinoa is cooking, place the artichoke hearts, sun-dried tomatoes, spinach or other greens, olive oil, garlic and chilli flakes in mixing bowl. When quinoa is finished, add it to the bowl, and then add a pinch of sea salt and goat's cheese, if desired.

Microwave No-Time Salmon with Broccoli

Servings: 1   **Cheats/Serving: 1.5**

1 frozen dinner with salmon that contains 100g of salmon
Frozen broccoli
Lemon juice to taste

Open the frozen dinner and discard any Cheat you don't want (rice, pasta, etc.). Open the broccoli and place it on top of your frozen dinner. Heat the salmon and broccoli until fully cooked, and then sprinkle with lemon juice.

Jerk Salmon

Servings: 4   **Cheats/Serving: 1.5**

As crazy as this sounds, if you're intimidated by the oven or saucepan, you can cook this in the microwave. I'll give you both the oven and microwave versions. Please do not get Atlantic farmed salmon for this recipe. Yes, it probably tastes better because it's fattier, but with these spices, you're really going to start liking wild salmon.

450g skinless, boneless salmon fillets
2 tbsp jerk seasoning
Sea salt and ground black pepper to taste

Oven directions:

Preheat the oven to 200°C/400°F/Gas Mark 6. Place salmon on parchment paper or foil, add the jerk spice, sea salt and ground black pepper. Wrap the fish into a package and place on a baking sheet. Bake for 20 minutes. (Depending on thickness, check after 15 minutes. It should easily come apart with a fork.)

Microwave directions:

Place salmon in microwave friendly dish (do not use plastic or metal). Add the jerk seasoning, sea salt, and ground black pepper. Cover with a lid or dish. Microwave for five minutes. Be careful, you might have a mess in your microwave if you don't cover it correctly, but sometimes it's worth not having to use the oven.

Bacon Avocado Burgers

Servings: 4   Cheats/Serving: 3

Serve these burgers with a large salad with Dijon or balsamic vinaigrette (remember, each portion is the large salad bowl that you usually serve for the family) or a baked sweet potato.

450g grass-fed minced beef, divided into 4 patties
1 tsp extra virgin olive oil
1 small onion, thinly sliced
450g button mushrooms
1 garlic clove, minced
Sea salt and ground black pepper to taste
4 servings bacon confetti (page 190)
1 avocado, sliced

Heat a large frying pan over a medium heat. Place the burger patties in the frying pan and cover. Monitor and flip the burgers every five minutes or so until cooked to your liking.

While the burgers are cooking, in large saucepan over medium heat, add the olive oil. Add the onions, mixing slowly. Do not leave the onions! Cook for around eight minutes, until the onions are medium amber in colour. Add the mushrooms and cook until they're lightly browned. Add the garlic, sea salt and ground black pepper and bacon confetti. (Two half strips are one Cheat.)

Salmon and Cucumber Wraps

Servings: 6   Cheats/Serving: 1

Juice of 1 lemon
450g smoked salmon
1 large cucumber, peeled
150g rocket, spinach or mixed greens
Capers (optional)

Squeeze lemon juice over the salmon. Using a vegetable peeler, thinly slice oblong pieces of cucumber. Next, place a slice of salmon and a bit of rocket inside the cucumber and add a few capers on top. Now wrap the cucumber around the salmon, greens and capers and place a toothpick through the bundle to hold it together. Repeat until you've used all your ingredients.

Tangy Tenderloin

Servings: 4 (with a 450g fillet)   Cheats/Serving: 3

120ml freshly squeezed lime juice
½ tsp coarse sea salt
¼ onion, finely chopped
3 garlic cloves, minced
100g honey
⅛ tsp ground black pepper
450g pork fillet
2 tbsp extra virgin olive oil

Mix all the ingredients except the oil and pork in a zip seal bag. Add the pork to the bag and coat well. Place in the refrigerator overnight, turning occasionally.

Preheat the oven to 220°C/425°F/Gas Mark 7. Remove the pork from the bag, discarding the remaining marinade.

Heat a frying pan over medium-high heat. Add the oil. Once the oil is hot, add the pork and sear each side until it's brown. Roast the pork in the oven for 15–20 minutes. Check to make sure it's fully cooked and serve.

Tasty Harissa Chicken

Servings: 4   **Cheats/Serving: 1.5**

½ tbsp extra virgin olive oil
450g chicken breast fillets
2 tbsp harissa spice
Sea salt and ground black pepper to taste
½ lime or lemon (optional)

Heat a saucepan over medium heat. Add oil and then add chicken. Sprinkle in the spice, sea salt, and ground black pepper, making sure to spread it evenly. Cook 8–10 minutes, flipping three to four times during cooking with tongs. Be sure to cut one piece of chicken open to ensure its cooked throughout (it's no longer dark pink). Squeeze ½ lime over the chicken if desired.

Tunatastic with Lemon and Garlic

Servings: 4   Cheats/Serving: 2

This is a great topping for mixed greens.

> *450g tinned tuna*
> *Juice of 1 large lemon*
> *1 tbsp extra virgin olive oil*
> *1 tsp balsamic vinegar*
> *1 garlic clove, minced*
> *Sea salt and ground black pepper to taste*

Add all the ingredients to a large bowl and mix well.

Cod with Baby Spinach, Tomatoes and Herbs

Servings: 4   Cheats/Serving: 1
                                          Cheat per 75g tilapia fillet

> *350g baby spinach*
> *Sea salt and ground black pepper to taste*
> *¼ tsp onion powder*
> *60ml home-made or low-sodium chicken broth*
> *4 x 75g skinless and boneless cod fillets*
> *4 spring onions, chopped*
> *2 tomatoes, chopped*

Preheat the oven to 180°C/350°F/Gas Mark 4.

Spray a baking dish with cooking spray or coat it with oil. Add the spinach to the baking dish, and then sprinkle it with sea salt, ground black pepper,and onion powder. Add the chicken broth.

Sprinkle the fish with sea salt and ground black pepper, and then place the fish on top of the spinach. Sprinkle with the spring onions.

Cover the baking dish with foil and bake for 20–25 minutes, or until the fish flakes easily with a fork.

Serve with the chopped tomatoes.

Wild Caught Fish with Olive Oil and Paprika Vegetables

Servings: 4   **Cheats/Serving: 1 cheat per 75g white fish fillet**

4 x 75g skinless and boneless white-fish fillets
2 white onions, sliced
350g fresh or frozen broccoli, cauliflower and carrot mix
Extra virgin olive oil
⅛ tsp paprika
Sea salt and ground black pepper to taste

Preheat the oven to 180°C/350°F/Gas Mark 4.

Cut four pieces of foil, each large enough to wrap one fish fillet. Place the fish on top of the foil. Add slices of onion and some of the vegetable mixture to the top of each fish. Drizzle each packet with olive oil and sprinkle with paprika, sea salt and ground black pepper.

Fold the foil into packets and place them on a baking sheet. Bake for 10–15 minutes.

Za'atar Grilled Chicken Strips

Servings: 4   **Cheats/Serving: 1.5**

½ tbsp extra virgin olive oil
450g chicken breast, precut
2 tbsp za'atar spice blend
½ tsp cayenne pepper
Sea salt and ground black pepper to taste

Heat a saucepan over medium heat. Add oil and then add chicken. Add Za'atar spice, cayenne pepper and sea salt and ground black pepper, making sure to spread it evenly. Cook 8–10 minutes, flipping three to four times during cooking with tongs. Be sure to cut one piece of chicken open to ensure its cooked throughout (it's no longer dark pink). These strips make a great addition to a salad.

Dinner Recipes

Soups

Best Cream of Spinach Soup

Servings: 8   **Cheats/Serving: 1**

400g coconut milk
600g frozen or fresh spinach
4 garlic cloves, chopped
Sea salt and ground black pepper to taste
Cayenne pepper or chilli flakes to taste
½ small glass of Chardonnay (optional)
½ apple, chopped (optional)

In a large saucepan over medium-high heat, add all the ingredients and bring it to a boil. Once boiling, remove from the heat. With a hand blender, blend the soup until it's smooth.

Black Bean and Salsa Short cut Soup

Servings: 6   **Cheats/Serving: 0, 1 if you do "Optionals"**

This can be a very easy recipe to make. If you look at any (good) black bean soup recipe, there is usually a long list vegetables and spices. By using salsa and a curry or spice mix like Madras Curry Powder, you can make this recipe very quickly.

Like any recipe we outline, there are many different directions you can take. We have outlined the base ingredients that you need to successfully make the recipe. We also outline a list of variable ingredients that you can use to customize the soup to match your tastes.

If you don't want bacon, can easily remove the bacon. If you have a family that includes men who wonder "where the real food is," you can up the bacon and maybe even add chunks of meat to make it more of a stew. This recipe includes plenty of nutrient-dense foods, serving the dual purpose of providing big doses of "good stuff" while also seeming like "real food."

Delivery is everything when introducing new healthy recipes and dinners in the home. When asked what's for dinner, if you answer black beans, salsa, and quinoa, invariably the answer becomes "Where's the beef?" or "That's bird food, how am I supposed to feel full?"

Always lead with the traditional ingredient. In this black bean soup, say, we're having bacon (or chicken or steak, whatever you've added). If everyone feels they are having a traditional protein, they don't anticipate dinners as this new healthy kick you're on, counting down the days until you revert back to spag bol. When you answer, "A new beef dish!" or "A special chicken hungry man chilli," they start to look forward to what's next.

400g dried black beans

750ml water

½ jalapeño or green chilli, finely chopped (onions are a nice replacement if you like flavour but not too much spice)

400g salsa

Madras curry paste or powder (or any favourite curry flavouring) to taste

Optional Ingredients

100g uncooked quinoa (or ½ –1 cup cooked if you already have it in your fridge)

2 bacon rashers

Chicken, beef or other protein, cut into large chunks

250g cooked and blended kale (Thanks to Jennifer Stewart for the suggestion on our Facebook page, who said, "You can't even tell the kale is in there.")

Any extra vegetables you want or have on hand, cut into large chunks

2 tbsp extra virgin olive oil, coconut oil or flaxseed oil (especially if you are an athlete)

Add the beans and water to a stockpot over a medium heat. Chop the chilli peppers (or onions) and add them to the water and the beans. Bring the mixture to a boil, and then add the salsa and curry powder. From here, this is really a "choose your own adventure" recipe. Add quinoa if you want to make a thicker soup or stew. Add some well-cooked bacon for some added flavour and texture. Add chicken or beef if that is a direction you want to head. Toss in vegetables or a couple tablespoons of oil. It's up to you.

Important Note: We strongly encourage you to follow Jennifer's suggestion and add blended kale. Kale and other greens are very high in nutrients that most of us don't get enough of. For example, kale contains the highest concentration of vitamin K of any food. Vitamin K is critical for bone health and healthy aging, yet experts say that poor intake of vitamin K is common.

We are focusing on this because: 1. The average adult eats very few greens; 2. Greens contain the highest concentration of vitamin K. Other excellent sources of vitamin K include spinach and Swiss chard.

Butternut Squash Soup

Servings: 8   **Cheats/Serving: 1**

(If using optional coconut milk,

0 if not)

The quality of the squash will make this soup just Ok or great. Look for dark skin and heavy weight for the size. Combine this soup with your favourite protein.

1 onion
1 tbsp extra virgin olive oil
1 medium to large butternut squash
1 apple
1.8l cold water
400ml coconut milk (optional)
1 tsp sea salt
Ground black pepper to taste (optional)
Fresh herbs (optional)
Lemon juice (optional)

Peel and cut the onion into quarters.

Heat a stockpot over a medium heat and add the oil. When it's hot, add the onion. While the onion browns, remove the skin of the squash and cut the squash into large pieces. Add the squash to the stockpot, letting it brown with the onion.

Peel and quarter the apple, and then add it to the pan. Add the water, coconut milk, and sea salt to the stockpot. Cook until everything is soft, about 30 minutes.

Blend with a hand blender until smooth. Garnish with ground black pepper, herbs and a squeeze of lemon juice, if desired.

Carrot Ginger Soup

Servings: 10   Cheats/Serving: 1

12 carrots, roughly chopped
1l chicken stock
1 bay leaf (optional)
400g coconut milk
1 large onion, chopped
1 tbsp extra virgin olive oil
5cm chunk fresh ginger, chopped
7 garlic cloves, minced
Juice of 2 limes
Crushed chilli flakes to taste
1 handful coriander, chopped
Sea salt to taste

Place the carrots, broth, bay leaf and coconut milk in a large stockpot over a high heat. Once boiling, turn down to a simmer.

In a large frying pan over a medium heat, sauté the onion in the olive oil until translucent and slightly soft and golden. Add the ginger and garlic and cook for just another minute or so. Add the onions, ginger and garlic into the stockpot.

After the mixture has come back to a boil, turn it down and simmer for 18 minutes. Remove the bay leaf and using hand blender, purée until smooth.

In a small saucepan, add the lime juice, chilli flakes, and coriander and cook over a high heat for a few minutes. Pour this mixture into the puréed soup and again use the hand blender to get the soup really smooth. Add sea salt to taste.

Chicken Pho Energy Soup

Servings: 8   **Cheats/Serving: 1**

This is a variation of the Energy Soup that we have been making for years. I add a bit of salad or spinach or whatever fresh greens I have in the fridge, but this is optional if you don't have them. Additionally, the greens really alter the flavour of the soup. For a more greens-based soup, definitely check out the Energy Soup recipe.

Pho broth *(you could use just chicken stock to save time)*
1l chicken stock
1 tbsp olive oil
1 onion chopped
5cm chunk fresh ginger, finely chopped
1 star anise
1 cardamom pod, peeled and crushed
1 tsp ground coriander
1 stick cinnamon
1tbsp soy sauce
1 tbsp fish sauce

½ a large head, fresh cauliflower
10 shiitake mushrooms (or use regular button mushrooms)
3 large heads of fresh broccoli (only ½ the stems)
400g coconut milk
5 shakes of chilli flakes (start with 2 shakes and increase from there to desired heat level)
½ tsp sea salt
Freshly ground black pepper to taste

If you're making the Pho broth, begin by frying the onion and ginger in a little oil. Add the spices and cook for a further minute before pouring in the stock. Bring to the boil then add the soy and fish sauce. Remove the star anise and cinnamon stick.

Add the coconut milk, cauliflower, mushrooms and broccoli to the stock or broth. Bring back to the boil then turn down the heat and simmer for 20 minutes. Add chilli flakes, sea salt and ground black pepper.

Using an hand blender, purée the soup. Taste for seasoning, and add more chilli flakes, sea salt, or ground black pepper as needed.

Cream of Broccoli Weight-Loss Cheat Cut Soup

Servings: 8   **Cheats/Serving: 1**

This soup travels wonderfully in a Thermos. Try it with the Italian Herb Goddess Chicken on page 237.

3 large broccoli heads (including stems)
5 garlic cloves
1l chicken or vegetable stock
400g coconut milk
225g fresh spinach leaves
½ jalapeño or green chilli, finely chopped (optional)
Sea salt and ground black pepper to taste (optional)

Cut the broccoli into quarters and mince the garlic.

Place the stock, coconut milk, broccoli, spinach, garlic, jalapeño, sea salt and ground black pepper in a large stockpot over high heat. When the mixture begins to boil, turn down the heat and simmer for 20 minutes.

With a hand blender, blend the soup until it's smooth. Taste, and add more sea salt and ground black pepper if needed.

Di's Hot Sausage Spice Soup

Servings: 6   **Cheats/Serving: 1**

"Di" is the fantastic mother of a dear friend. Her gourmet soups are often the highlight of the dinner party.

200g spicy chorizo, sliced
3 tbsp basil
2 tbsp garlic, chopped
3 tbsp fresh oregano
1 tbsp chilli flakes
3 spring onions, chopped
1 carrot, chopped
½ head savoy cabbage (or more if you'd like)
800ml chicken or beef stock
1 small green pepper
150g sliced mushrooms
300g potatoes, peeled and diced
120g tomato purée

Place the chopped chorizo in a stockpot over a medium heat. Once the oils being to release add the basil, garlic, oregano, chilli flakes and spring onions and stir. Add the carrot, cabbage and all the other ingredients. Bring to a boil, then turn down the heat and simmer for 20 minutes.

Serve with home-made garlic and cheese croutons.

Di's Lentil Soup

Servings: 8   Cheats/Serving: 0

1 tbsp extra virgin olive oil
1 carrot, chopped
1 celery stalk, chopped
1 small onion, chopped
1–3 garlic cloves, minced
3 tomatoes, chopped
1 tsp bouillon powder
200g lentils rinsed (green or red; I like green)
800ml chicken or vegetable broth, or water
900g fresh or frozen spinach
Sea salt and ground black pepper to taste
Chilli flakes (optional)
Cheese for topping (optional)

In a stockpot, heat the olive oil over medium heat. Add the carrot, celery, onion, garlic, tomatoes and bouillon powder and then fry for one minute.

Add the lentils and broth and bring to a boil. Turn the heat down to low.

Cover and cook for 30 minutes. Add the spinach and cook uncovered for 20 minutes. Add sea salt, ground black pepper and chilli flakes. Cook for 10 more minutes. Serve topped with cheese.

The Famous Puréed Energy Soup

Servings: 10   **Cheats/Serving: 1**

People call and write to me almost every day to tell me that they lose weight when they add this soup to their diet. If you are trying to lose weight, eat this soup before you eat other foods.

Note that unless you use a hand blender, this recipe will be a big pain and you won't be as likely to do it.

A few suggested pairings for this soup: black beans (toss them right into the soup), extra firm tofu (fry it for five minutes with a bit of olive oil, sesame seeds and chilli flakes) or 100g of baked salmon or other protein.

1l chicken or vegetable stock
400g coconut milk
3 stalks of broccoli (cut off the stalk ends)
450g bag frozen or fresh spinach (fresh gives it a beautiful spring green colour)
250g mushrooms (shiitake or a mixed box)
6 carrots
2 fresh bay leaves
1 medium onion, chopped
1 tbsp extra virgin olive oil
10cm chunk of fresh ginger, roughly chopped
6 medium garlic cloves
Juice of 2–3 fresh limes to taste
Crushed chilli flakes to taste
1 handful fresh coriander, chopped
Sea salt to taste

In a large stockpot over high heat, add the chicken broth and coconut milk and then add the broccoli, spinach, mushrooms, carrots and bay leaves. Bring to a boil, then turn down the heat and simmer for 18–20 minutes.

In a separate saucepan or large frying pan over medium heat, sauté the onions in olive oil until they are slightly soft and browned. Be careful not to burn them.

In a food processor, grind the ginger and garlic, and then stir them into the onions and cook for a minute. Add the onion mixture to the broth in the stockpot.

In same pan in which you sautéed the onions, place lime juice, crushed chilli flakes and the coriander. Fry the mixture over a high heat for 1–2 minutes. Add this mixture to the large stockpot.

Using a hand blender, purée the soup until smooth. It should be a bit thick, which will help keep you satiated. Taste and add sea salt as needed. You can also add a bit more lime, chilli flakes or coriander as needed.

Herbed Beef and Bacon Soup

Servings: 6   **Cheats/Serving: 2.5**

450g grass-fed minced beef
225g organic bacon, cooked and crumbled
400g tinned, chopped tomatoes
1 onion, chopped
2 celery stick, chopped
300ml beef stock
300g mixed vegetables, chopped (carrots, root vegetables, spinach,
   chard, cabbage, kale)
⅛ tbsp dried rosemary
⅛ tbsp dried thyme
¼ tsp dried basil
Sea salt and ground black pepper to taste

Add all the ingredients to a slow cooker. Cook on low heat for five hours, or until the minced beef is thoroughly cooked.

Home-made Chicken Stock

Servings: 8 to 12   **Cheats/Serving: 0.5 per 250ml**

This broth is wonderful for freezing so it's available whenever a recipe calls for chicken stock.

1 whole chicken
1 onion, chopped
4 celery stalks, chopped into 10cm pieces
4 carrots, chopped into 10cm pieces
½ garlic bulb, cloves peeled

Place the chicken in a slow cooker and cover with cold water. Add the remaining ingredients.

Cook on low heat for eight hours, or until the meat is tender. Separate the meat from the bones, leaving everything in the slow cooker.

Place a colander in a large bowl, and then pour the stock from the slow cooker into the colander to separate the liquid from the solids.

Insane Man Hunger Chilli

Servings: 3   **Cheats/Serving: 1**

When you travel or are on the go, make a mix of this and put it in containers. Salsa is the secret ingredient for this chilli because it contains everything you need to make the recipe super tasty, but all you have to do is open the container into the pot! We find that the hottest salsa provides the most flavour, and dissipates once among the other ingredients.

A note on the meat: you can add more meat if you'd like, but we strongly advise spending a little more for higher quality meat. A little goes a long way, and you're getting plenty of protein from other sources. Organic beef doesn't have antibiotics or added hormones. Most lamb is grass fed and a 500g portion will cost about four pounds. Remember, as the quality of meat goes down, so does the price. For vegetarians and vegans, there are a whole host of replacement items you could use, which you already know about and love. Choose your favourite for this chilli.

1 onion (optional – there are some onions already in the ready-made salsa)
Fresh ginger, finely chopped (optional)
4–6 garlic cloves, smashed (optional)
Curry powder to taste (optional)
225g grass-fed lamb or beef
300g salsa
800g tinned kidney beans, drained and rinsed
225g chopped greens (Fresh spinach works great, but you can also use frozen greens here: spinach, kale, endive, whatever you have.)

If using extra onions, ginger, garlic or curry, heat a little oil in your pot over medium heat, and then add the optional ingredients and fry just until the onion starts to brown.

This mix is a very powerful combination that has been shown to help fight all sorts of really nasty diseases.

Once the onion is browned, or if you are not using the optional ingredients, add your meat and the salsa, and mix together. Once it has started to cook, add the drained and rinsed beans. Mix it around. After three minutes, put the greens in, turn down the heat a touch and cover the pot. Let it simmer for a couple more minutes.

The greens cook almost instantly and the beans heat up quickly. The key is to make sure the meat thoroughly cooks.

Feel free to add more greens if you wish. You can serve this over quinoa or with other vegetables.

Orr's Island Vegetable Soup

Servings: 4   **Cheats/Serving: 0**

Our kitchen is seldom without a pot of vegetable soup made from whatever vegetables happen to look fresh in the market. My mother-in-law plays around with this recipe depending on what is available. You can add cooked chickpeas, white beans or any other kind of bean to make it a meal.

This soup is also perfect for your slow cooker. Cook it on high for about four hours or on low for 5–6 hours, depending on your cooker.

Some of the vegetables that go into the soup include chayote (pear-shaped pale green) and butternut squash. Chayote (pronounced Chai-o-tay), is also known as the vegetable pear, mirliton, or christophene and is originally native to Mexico and Central America. Though mild and almost bland in taste, it is packed with nutrients and rich in amino acids and vitamin C. The leaves and fruit have diuretic, cardiovascular, and anti-inflammatory properties, and a tea made from the leaves has been used in the treatment of arteriosclerosis and hypertension, and to dissolve kidney stones.

2l of chicken stock
2 carrots, cut into chunks
1 onion, thickly sliced
4–5 garlic cloves, peeled and chopped
1 tsp chopped fresh ginger (optional)
Dash of turmeric powder (optional)
1 large tomato, cut into chunks
1 jalapeño or green chilli, finely chopped (more or less to your taste)
150g butternut squash, cut into chunks
1 chayote (Christophene), cut into chunks (you could use courgette instead)
½ cabbage, roughly chopped
1 handful spinach, Swiss chard or other leafy green
Juice of 1 lime or ½ lemon
Fresh coriander, chopped

In a large stockpot bring the stock to a boil. Add the carrots, onion, garlic, ginger, turmeric, and tomatoes, and simmer over medium heat for 6–7minutes.

Add the jalapeños, squash and chayote (or courgette), and simmer until the vegetables are almost cooked. Add the cabbage and leafy greens, and cook for another few minutes.

Turn off the heat and add the lime or lemon juice. Garnish with coriander.

Cleanse Soup

Servings: 10   **Cheats/Serving: 1**

1 tbsp extra virgin olive oil
1 large onion chopped
650g white button mushrooms, sliced
900ml chicken or vegetable stock
400g coconut milk
2 large heads broccoli, chopped
1 large head cauliflower, chopped
450g spinach (optional)
2 fingers' worth of fresh ginger, peeled
1 finger's worth of fresh turmeric, peeled
5 garlic cloves, crushed
Sea salt to taste

Heat a stockpot over medium heat. Add the oil, and once it's warm, add the onion to the pot.

Brown the onions, stirring constantly. Once they're light brown, add the mushrooms and continue to cook until the mushrooms are light brown.

Add the broth and coconut milk, and then turn the heat up to high. Add the broccoli, cauliflower, spinach, ginger, turmeric and garlic and bring to a boil. Turn the heat down and simmer for 15 minutes.

Let the soup stand for 10 minutes before using a hand blender to blend the soup until smooth. Taste and add sea salt as needed.

Spicy Pumpkin Ginger Soup

Servings: 10 to 12   **Cheats/Serving: 1**

This soup is a Thanksgiving staple in our home. Served by the fireside as a first course, it never fails to wow guests. That said, there's no reason you couldn't serve it chilled in the summertime as well.

2 tbsp extra virgin olive oil
1 large onion, finely chopped
2 garlic cloves, minced
1 small potato, boiled, peeled, and cubed
1½ tbsp ginger, minced
⅛ tsp ground cardamom
¼ tsp freshly grated nutmeg
1 tbsp curry powder
¾ tsp cayenne ground black pepper (or more to taste)
1l chicken or vegetable stock
Sea salt to taste
800g tinned pumpkin purée
500ml water
400g coconut milk
2 tbsp coriander, chopped
1 jalapeño or green chilli finely chopped
Juice of ½ lemon
1 tbsp ginger, finely julienned

In a large stockpot over medium heat, add the olive oil. Once it's hot, add the onions. Cook, stirring occasionally, until softened, about five minutes. Add the garlic, potato, and ginger and continue cooking for a minute, stirring constantly.

Add the spices, and then purée in a blender or food processor with a little stock. Return to the pot. Add the sea salt, pumpkin, water, the remaining stock and coconut milk, stirring to combine, and simmer gently, uncovered, for about 20 minutes.

TNT's Veggie Weight-Loss Soup

Servings: 12   **Cheats/Serving: 0.5**

This recipe is from someone who did not like my soup, so she made her own! It's best when it's served piping hot. The possibilities for this soup are endless – leave out vegetables you don't like or add in those you do. Substitute brown rice or quinoa for the lentils.

400g of lentils
2–3 courgettes, sliced and quartered
200g chestnut mushrooms
6 celery stalks, sliced
Garlic powder to taste
1.5l chicken or vegetable stock
800g frozen stir-fry vegetables
250g frozen, chopped spinach
450g frozen, crinkle cut carrots
450g frozen, cut green beans
450g frozen, baby broccoli florets
Cayenne to taste
Ground black pepper to taste

Cook the lentils according to packet instructions (usually one part lentils to one part water).

In a large stockpot, combine the courgette, mushrooms and celery. Sprinkle with garlic powder, stir and add a cup or so of stock. Cook over a high heat until the courgette and celery s tart to become translucent. Be careful not to overcook the vegetables. Turn off the heat, but leave the pot on the stove. Add the stir-fry vegetables.

One by one, microwave the frozen vegetables (as per individual cooking instructions), and then add them to the stockpot.

Add all the remaining stock and the cooked lentils. Stir gently with a big spoon. Lastly, sprinkle with cayenne and ground black pepper and stir again.

Warm Applewood Bacon Soup

Servings: 4   **Cheats/Serving: .5**

This is one of our most popular soups!

2 rashers applewood bacon (or any smoked bacon)
3 medium garlic cloves, minced or pressed
1 medium sweet onion, thinly sliced into 5cm strips
1 head of cauliflower, chopped into 5cm pieces
800ml chicken stock
1 tsp rosemary, finely chopped
225g fresh spinach leaves
1–2 squeezes of fresh lemon juice
Sea salt and freshly ground black pepper to taste

In a large frying pan, cook the bacon over medium-low heat until it's crisp. Use tongs to take out the bacon and place it on paper towels. Drain most of the bacon grease, leaving just a little to cook the rest of the ingredients in.

Add the garlic, onion and cauliflower to the frying pan, stir over a medium heat until the cauliflower and onion start to turn golden brown. Add the chicken stock, rosemary and spinach, and cook until the cauliflower and spinach are tender, anywhere from 5–10 minutes.

Remove the pan from the heat. Chop the cooked bacon and return it to the pan, add the lemon juice and season to taste.

Warm Cream of Tomato Soup

Servings: 8   **Cheats/Serving: 1**

400g coconut milk
1.2kg chopped tomatoes (about 3 tins)
3 garlic cloves, minced
Sea salt and ground black pepper to taste

Place a pot over a high heat. Add all the ingredients, and bring to a boil. Once boiling, turn the heat down and let it simmer just for a minute or two. With a hand blender, blend the soup until smooth.

Weight Loss Short cut Soup

Servings: 8   **Cheats/Serving: 1**

This soup travels wonderfully in a Thermos. Try it with the Italian Herb Goddess Chicken on page 237.

3 large broccoli heads (including stems)
5 garlic cloves
900ml chicken or vegetable stock
400g coconut milk
225g fresh spinach leaves
½ jalapeño or green chilli finely chopped (optional)
Sea salt and ground black pepper to taste (optional)

Cut the broccoli into quarters and mince the garlic.

Place the stock, coconut milk, broccoli, spinach, garlic, jalapeño, sea salt, and ground black pepper in a large stockpot over high heat. When the mixture begins to boil, turn down the heat and simmer for 20 minutes. With a hand blender, blend the soup until it's smooth. Taste season as needed.

Slow Cooker and Stews

Classic Pork Loin Roast Tacos

Servings: 12   **Cheats/Serving: 2**

1.5kg boneless pork loin, cubed (or shoulder of pork)
½ tsp sea salt
Ground black pepper
2 green chilli peppers, finely chopped
3 garlic cloves, minced
800ml water
125g chipotle sauce
1 head of lettuce, quartered

Place the pork in a slow cooker and cover with the sea salt, ground black pepper, chilli and garlic, and then pour 125ml of water and the chipotle sauce on top.

Cover and cook on low for six hours. Remove the pork from the slow cooker and with two forks, shred the pork.

Return the meat to the slow cooker and allow it to sit in the juices for 15 minutes.

Serve wrapped in lettuce leaves.

Dad's Hearty Beef Stew

Servings: 8   **Cheats/Serving: 3**

900g stewing beef, cut into 2.5cm chunks
2 large carrots, chopped
2 sticks celery, chopped
3 medium onions, chopped
5 tbsp extra virgin olive oil
5 tbsp almond flour or almond meal

400g tomato passata
250ml low-salt beef stock

Add all the ingredients to a slow cooker. Cook on medium heat 4–6 hours, or until the beef is tender.

New Orleans Chicken and Sausage Gumbo

Servings: 6   **Cheats/Serving: 1**

Try this over brown cauliflower rice (page 255) or steamed broccoli.

120g boneless, skinless, free-range chicken breasts, cubed
120g cooked, smoked sausage, chopped
2 celery stalks with leaves, sliced
1 large carrot, chopped
1 medium onion
400g tinned, chopped tomatoes
1.25l water
1 tsp thyme
300g frozen or fresh okra, thawed, drained and cut

Mix all the ingredients, except the okra, into a slow cooker. Cover and cook on low heat for 6.5–7 hours. Stir in the okra and cook for 20 more minutes.

Slow Cooker Chicken and Spinach Soup

Servings: 4   **Cheats/Serving: 2**

You could make a quick version of this using leftover roasted chicken or cooked breast pieces.

450g chicken, cut into bite-sized pieces
450g fresh spinach
2 onions, diced

2 tsp chilli flakes (optional)
Sea salt and ground black pepper to taste
900ml chicken stock

In a slow cooker, add all the ingredients and stir. Simmer on a low heat for three hours. Watch while it's cooking in case more stock or water is needed. Adjust seasonings before serving.

Slow Cooker Clean-Eating Cheat-Free Soup

Servings: 4   **Cheats/Serving: 0**

1 carrot, chopped
1 large onion, chopped
1 tbsp extra virgin olive oil
400g tinned, chopped tomatoes
180g chopped cabbage
1 tsp sea salt
¼ tsp ground black pepper
150g dried butter beans
1 large handful of flat-leaf parsley, chopped
500ml water or coconut water

Add all the ingredients to a slow cooker. Cook on a medium heat for 3–4 hours, or until the beans are soft.

Slow Cooker Fire-Roasted Tomato Beef Chilli

Servings: 8   **Cheats/Serving: 2**

1kg stewing beef, cut into 2.5cm chunks
1 large onion, diced
200g mushrooms, sliced
2 medium carrots, chopped
2 tbsp chilli powder
1 tsp cumin

1 tsp garlic salt
800g tinned, chopped tomatoes
800g fire-roasted tomato sauce or soup
½ tsp oregano
1 tbsp extra virgin olive oil
800ml water
2 tsp sea salt (optional)

Add all the ingredients to a slow cooker. Cook on medium heat for 4–6 hours, until the beef is thoroughly cooked.

Slow Cooker Garlic and Paprika Roasted Chicken

Servings: 16 to 20   **Cheats/Serving: 2**

This recipe works best with a chicken that has a pop-up timer.

1.8kg–2.25kg whole fresh chicken
120ml extra virgin olive oil
2 tsp paprika
4 garlic gloves, minced
Sea salt and ground black pepper to taste

Prep the chicken by cleaning out the cavity so no innards are left (most supermarket chickens already have the giblets removed). Rub hardened coconut oil all over the chicken, and then rub paprika, garlic, sea salt and ground black pepper all over the chicken, both inside and out.

Place the chicken in a slow cooker. Cook on high for an hour, and then reduce the heat to low and cook an additional five hours until the meat is tender.

Slow Cooker Wraps

Servings: varies   **Cheats/Serving: varies based on the protein**

Leftover protein or casserole from the slow cooker
Large cabbage leaves

Add leftovers to the large cabbage leaves, wrapping the leaf around the leftovers. If you want to transport this, wrap foil around the cabbage leaf.

Oven Baked and Casseroles

Brian's Sweet Potato and Coconut Meatballs

Servings: 4 (4–6 meatballs each)   **Cheats/Serving: 2**

Brian Rigby is a performance nutrition expert who runs a thriving practice in Boulder, USA.

Brian says, "When I can find 95 per cent lean, grass-fed minced beef on sale, I'll make up some meatballs (or hamburgers, depending on my whim). I tend to be a little random in what I put into them, but here's a recipe I'll use from time to time. The sweet potato keeps the meatballs moist, which is useful because the extra-lean beef doesn't have a lot of fat!"

450g lean, grass-fed minced beef
1 large (250g) sweet potato, grated
30g unsweetened shredded coconut
4–8 garlic cloves, minced (I love garlic, but not everybody is as in love with it as I am...use less if you want!)
1 tsp ground black pepper
Cayenne pepper to taste
Sea salt to taste

Preheat the oven to 200°C/400°F/Gas Mark 6. Line a baking sheet with parchment paper. Mix the beef, sweet potato, coconut, garlic, ground black pepper, cayenne pepper and sea salt in a bowl. Form meatballs 2–3cm in diameter and place on the lined baking sheet.

Bake the meatballs for 30–35 minutes, or until browned on the outside and no longer pink on the inside.

These can be served any way you'd normally serve meatballs, or you can toss them in a soup or on a salad for an easy protein option.

Chicken Bake

Servings: 8   **Cheats/Serving: 1.5**

4 boneless, skinless, free-range chicken breasts
Sea salt and ground black pepper to taste
1 tbsp extra virgin olive oil
4 medium carrots, thinly sliced
2 medium courgettes, thinly sliced
12 mushrooms, thinly sliced
4 spring onions, thinly sliced
2 thumb's worth of ginger, minced
4 tbsp tamari or light soy sauce

Preheat the oven to 200°C/400°F/Gas Mark 6.

Cut four pieces of parchment paper, each large enough to wrap each chicken breast and a quarter of the vegetables. Season the chicken breasts with sea salt and ground black pepper. Place one breast on each piece of parchment paper.

Drizzle olive oil over each chicken breast. Add a quarter of the vegetables and one tablespoon of tamari to each packet. Loosely wrap each chicken breast and vegetable mixture with the parchment paper.

Place the packets on an oven tray and bake 30–35 minutes, or until the chicken is thoroughly cooked (there should be no pink left when the chicken is cut open).

Chicken, Artichoke, Mushroom with Parmesan Casserole

Servings: 8   **Cheats/Serving: 2**

This mushroom mixture is a great addition to any traditional protein like grilled chicken, or on top of a bed of mixed greens.

900g chicken breast

Mushroom Mixture
250g mushrooms
225g cherry tomatoes
6 garlic cloves
1 large handful of coriander
250g artichoke hearts, quartered and rinsed
4 tbsp extra virgin olive oil
Juice of ½ lemon
Sea salt and ground black pepper to taste
1–2 tsp chilli flakes (or more to taste)
450g spinach
Goat's cheese or Parmesan confetti (optional)

Preheat the oven to 180°C/350°F/Gas Mark 4.

Heat a frying pan over a medium heat. Once hot, brown the chicken breast on all sides. While the chicken is browning, prepare the mushroom mixture.

Slice the mushrooms into small pieces, about 4–5 per mushroom. Slice the cherry tomatoes in half. Grind the garlic cloves and chop the coriander leaves, throwing the stems away.

In a large mixing bowl, mix the mushrooms, tomatoes, garlic, coriander, artichoke hearts, olive oil and the lemon juice. Add the sea salt, ground black pepper and chilli flakes.

Line the bottom of a casserole dish with the spinach then place the browned chicken breast on top. Add the mushroom mixture on top of the chicken, and finish with goat's cheese or Parmesan confetti. Bake for 30 minutes.

Coconut Chicken Tenders

Servings: 3   **Cheats/Serving: 3**

Serve these chicken tenders with fresh vegetables.

30g walnuts
30g almonds
7 tbsp shredded unsweetened coconut
⅛ tsp sea salt
3 egg whites
6 free-range chicken breast fillets
⅛ tsp ground black pepper
⅛ tsp garlic powder

Preheat the oven to 190°C/375°F/Gas Mark 5.

In a food processor, grind the walnuts and almonds. Add the ground nuts to a bowl and mix in the coconut flakes, garlic powder, ground black pepper and sea salt. In a separate bowl, whisk the egg whites.

Coat a baking dish with non-stick cooking spray or line the dish with parchment paper.

Dip the chicken into the egg whites and then into the coconut mixture. Place the chicken in the baking dish.

Bake for 25–30 minutes, turning once, halfway through. The chicken is done when it is no longer pink in the centre and the coconut is golden brown.

Cold Winter's Night Casserole

Servings: 8   **Cheats/Serving: 2**

2 aubergines
1 tsp sea salt, plus some for sprinkling on the aubergine
1–2 onions, diced
2 tbsp extra virgin olive oil
1 potato, thinly sliced
450g minced lamb
½ tsp ground black pepper
1 large splash of red wine
1 large splash of chicken stock
¼ tsp chilli flakes
1 tsp cinnamon
1 tomato, chopped
1 small tin of tomato sauce
3 tbsp chopped parsley
125ml water
Parmesan cheese

Topping
1 tbsp butter
1 tbsp olive oil
2 tbsp flour
400g coconut milk
¼ tsp of sea salt
⅛ tsp ground white pepper
4–5 grates of fresh nutmeg

Preheat the oven to 190°C/375°F/Gas Mark 5.

Slice the aubergine thinly. Sprinkle with sea salt and allow the juices to drain away in a colander for 30 minutes. Squeeze the juices out, rinse with cold water and pat dry. Fry each slice lightly in a non-stick pan and place to one side.

Fry the onions in the olive oil until golden. Add the potato and fry for a few minutes. Add the minced lamb, sea salt and ground black pepper, and fry until brown. Add the red wine and allow it to reduce down a little. Then add the chicken stock and chilli flakes. Add the cinnamon, chopped tomato, tomato sauce, parsley and water. Simmer for 15 minutes until the water is absorbed.

In a lasagne dish, alternate the layers of aubergine slices and meat mixture, topping every other layer with a sprinkling of Parmesan cheese.

To make the topping, melt the butter in the saucepan and add the olive oil. Add the flour and stir over a low heat for a few minutes until well blended. When the flour smells slightly nutty, add the coconut milk gradually, stirring until it boils. Use a whisk so lumps do not form. Season with sea salt, white pepper and fresh nutmeg. Simmer until the sauce thickens. Pour the sauce over the aubergine and meat mixture and bake, uncovered, for 45 minutes. Cut into squares to serve.

Favourite Roast Chicken

Servings: 8   **Cheats/Serving: 2**

Tip: Make this chicken on a beer can chicken roaster. You can find them online and they can be used for any chicken dish you cook.

2 tsp hot paprika
2 tsp onion powder
2 tsp garlic powder
1 tbsp extra virgin olive oil
1 tsp sea salt
1 tsp ground black pepper
1 whole chicken

Preheat the oven to 200°C/400°F/Gas Mark 6.

Mix together the spices, oil, sea salt and ground black pepper.

Slather the spice mixture all over the chicken. Place the chicken on the beer can roaster and roast for 1 hour and 45 minutes.

Let it rest for 20 minutes before eating so all the juices go back into the bird.

Hearty Meatloaf Muffins

Servings: 8   **Cheats/Serving: 2**

This recipe makes a lot of servings, but they freeze well for easy meals later!

900g minced beef
2 red onions, finely chopped
4 garlic cloves, minced
½ red pepper, finely chopped
1 handful coriander, chopped
1 handful parsley, chopped
2 tsp cumin
1 tsp ground black pepper
3 omega-3 enriched eggs

Preheat the oven to 190°C/375°F/Gas Mark 5.

Add all the ingredients to a zip seal food storage bag, and mash together until it's well mixed.

Scoop out the mixture into muffin tins, and then bake for 45 minutes.

Hot Italian Salmon Garlic Scampi

Servings: 4   Cheats/Serving: 2

People say that this tastes like Italian shrimp scampi (not the breaded kind!) but without the pasta and shrimp! With six ingredients and six minutes of prep time, make a dish I've never had anyone dislike.

Fresh salmon is the key to this recipe. If it isn't fresh, it just doesn't taste as good.

Juice of 1 lemon
450g fresh salmon
1½ tbsp extra virgin olive oil
7 garlic cloves, fresh and crushed (enough to cover the
*   salmon completely!)*
10 shakes chilli flakes
Sea salt

Preheat the oven to 200°C/400°F/Gas Mark 6.

In a large casserole dish, place a large piece of foil large enough to wrap completely around the salmon. Squeeze a bit of fresh lemon juice on the foil so the salmon doesn't stick.

Place the salmon in the dish and drizzle olive oil on top. Then squeeze the remaining lemon juice over the fish. Add the garlic, chilli flakes and sea salt, being sure to spread everything evenly over the salmon. Seal the foil.

Place in the oven for 28 minutes, and then use a knife to check if it's cooked – the fish should flake easily. It will most likely need 5 –10 minutes more (33–38 minutes total), depending on your oven. Try not to overcook the fish.

Any leftover salmon makes a great protein for other meals.

Italian Herb Goddess Chicken

Servings: 2   **Cheats/Serving: 1.5**

Serve this chicken with the Cream of Broccoli Weight-Loss Cheat Cut Soup on page 210.

---

2 boneless, skinless chicken breasts (100g each)
1 tbsp extra virgin olive oil
Sea salt and ground black pepper to taste
1 lemon, sliced
1 lime, sliced
1 handful fresh herbs (basil and oregano are favourites)

Preheat the oven to 180°C/350°F/Gas Mark 4.

Rub the chicken breast with oil, sea salt and ground black pepper. In a baking dish, place a piece of foil large enough to wrap the chicken.

Place the chicken on the foil and lay the lemon and lime slices on top. Rinse the fresh herbs and lay on top as well. Fold the foil over the chicken and seal the edges.

Bake for 25–35 minutes.

Japanese Chilli Salmon

Servings: 4   **Cheats/Serving: 2**

This salmon makes great leftovers to accompany other meals.

450g skinless and boneless salmon fillets
1 tbsp extra virgin olive oil
1 tsp fresh sesame seeds
4 shakes chilli flakes or cayenne pepper (to taste)
Sea salt

Preheat the oven to 200°C/400°F/Gas Mark 6. In a large casserole dish, place a piece of foil large enough to wrap the salmon.

Place the salmon on the foil and drizzle with the olive oil. Add the sesame seeds, chilli flakes or cayenne and sea salt, being sure to spread everything evenly over the salmon. Seal the foil around the salmon. Bake for 25 minutes.

Lemon Herb Salmon

Servings: 4   **Cheats/Serving: 2**

2 lemons
½ tbsp extra virgin olive oil
1 garlic clove, minced
Sea salt and ground black pepper to taste
450g skinless and boneless salmon fillets
1 handful of fresh dill, chopped

Preheat the oven to 220°C/425°F/Gas Mark 7. Line a baking sheet with foil or parchment paper, big enough to wrap the salmon.

Cut one lemon in slices and one lemon in quarters (to get the juice). Combine the olive oil, garlic and lemon juice from the quartered lemon in a small bowl with sea salt and pepper.

Place the fish on the foil or parchment paper and spread the lemon mixture evenly over the fish. Sprinkle the chopped dill all over and around the fish (use all your dill!) and then top with the lemon slices. Seal the parchment paper or foil to completely enclose the salmon is inside.

Cook for 10 minutes or until the salmon flakes with a fork. You can serve with more lemon slices if you want.

Mint and Shallot Halibut with Kale and Oven-Roasted Tomatoes

Servings: 4

Cheats/Serving: 1.5

450g tomatoes
1 tbsp extra virgin olive oil
450g halibut
2 mint sprigs
5 tbsp shallot, minced
450g kale
125ml vegetable stock

Preheat the oven to 220°C/425°F/Gas Mark 7.

Depending on the size of your tomatoes, either roughly chop them or halve them. Spread the tomatoes out evenly on a baking sheet, and then drizzle with the olive oil. Bake for 25–30 minutes.

While the tomatoes are baking, place a piece of foil large enough to wrap the fish into an baking dish. Add the halibut to the middle of the foil, and then evenly distribute the mint and shallot over the fish. Wrap the foil tightly around the fish. When the tomatoes have about 10 minutes left, add the fish to the oven. Everything should be done about the same time – just make sure the fish is opaque.

Remove the stems from the kale, and then roughly chop the leaves. In a large saucepan over a medium heat, add the vegetable stock. Once the stock is simmering, add the kale and cook until it's wilted.

To serve, place a bed of kale on the bottom of your plate, add the tomatoes then the halibut on top.

Poisson en Papillote

Servings: 8   **Cheats/Serving: 1.5 per 100g serving**

100ml freshly squeezed lemon juice
½ tsp sea salt
¼ onion, finely chopped
3 garlic cloves, minced
⅛ tsp paprika
⅛ tsp ground black pepper
4 x 200g wild-caught Alaskan salmon fillets
1 fresh lemon, quartered

Add all the ingredients except the salmon and lemon quarters to a zip seal food storage bag. Seal the bag and shake to mix.

Add the salmon to the bag and shake it to make sure each fillet is well coated. Refrigerate overnight, turning occasionally.

Preheat the oven to 220°C/425°F/Gas Mark 7.

Cut eight sheets of parchment paper, each measuring 30cm by 40cm (each fillet gets 2 sheets). Fold each one in half crosswise, then open and lay them flat.

Remove the salmon from the bag and discard the remaining marinade. Lay each fillet on one side of the parchment paper. Fold the paper over the salmon, making small, overlapping pleats as you go along to create a half-moon shape (similar to a Cornish pasty). Place the parcels on a baking dish. Bake for 8 minutes. Serve with a lemon wedge.

Sesame and Honey Chicken

Servings: 8   **Cheats/Serving: 3**

Serve this chicken with Cheat-Free Stir-fry (page 244) or cauliflower rice (page 255).

250g honey
6 tbsp tamari or light soy sauce
4 boneless, skinless, free-range chicken breasts
150g sesame seeds

Preheat the oven to 180°C/350°F/Gas Mark 4.

In a zip seal food storage bag, add the honey, tamari and chicken. Mix well, completely coating the chicken.

Remove the chicken from the bag and bake on a oven tray for 10 minutes.

Meanwhile, add the sesame seeds to a mixing bowl. Remove the chicken from the oven and coat well with the sesame seeds.

Return the chicken to the oven for 10 more minutes, or until the chicken is no longer pink in the centre.

Shepherd's Pie

Servings: 10   **Cheats/Serving: 3**

4 tbsp extra virgin olive oil
1 large onion, chopped
450g grass-fed or nitrate-free bacon, chopped
2 medium carrots, diced
2 celery stalks, diced
450g grass-fed minced beef
½ tsp sea salt

1 tsp freshly ground black pepper
250ml chicken stock
2 large heads of cauliflower, chopped

Preheat the oven to 180°C/350°F/Gas Mark 4.

Heat two tablespoons of the olive oil in a large frying pan over medium heat. Sauté the onion until it's soft and browned, about 15 minutes.

Add the bacon and cook for 10 minutes. Add the carrots and celery and cook an additional 10 minutes.

Add the minced beef and cook until it's brown. Mix in the sea salt and ground black pepper. Add the chicken stock and bring it to a simmer, cooking until the stock has reduced by 60 per cent.

Meanwhile, in a saucepan bring about 5cm of water to boil to cook the cauliflower. (You could use a steamer basket inside the saucepan instead.) Cover and cook until the cauliflower is soft, about 10 minutes.

Drain the cauliflower and add it to a food processor or blender. Add the remaining 2 tbsp of olive oil and process until smooth.

Pour the beef mixture into a baking dish, and then layer the cauliflower on top. Sprinkle with extra bacon bits if desired.

Bake for 30 minutes.

Protein Based (tradition and lean)

Servings: 4   **Cheats/Serving: 2**

Arroz Con Pollo

3 peppers (as many different colours as you can)
2 onions, chopped
200g broccoli (sounds strange but is delicious!)
450g chicken breast, cut into bite-sized pieces
Cayenne pepper to taste
Adobo or peri peri seasoning to taste
½ tbsp extra virgin olive oil
2 garlic cloves, chopped
Chopped jalapeños or green chillies to taste (optional)
60g green olives (optional)
125ml chicken stock
250ml water
125g cooked rice (Mexican rice is best)
1 handful coriander, chopped

Dice the bell ground black peppers, onions and broccoli. Coat the chicken breasts in cayenne and adobo seasoning. Word to the wise: less cayenne pepper is more for those who don't like it hot; you can never put too much adobo on chicken.

Put a large saucepan (that you have a lid for) on the stove over a medium heat. When the pan is hot, add the olive oil. Once that's hot add the garlic, onions and jalapeños. Cook these until the onions are almost translucent, about three minutes. Add the chicken breast and cook until the outsides are white but the chicken is not fully cooked, about three minutes. Add olives if you are using them (a little of the juice from the jar is also delicious in this recipe). Add the stock and simmer for 2–3 minutes. Add the vegetables and water, then cover so that the mixture can steam. Check every five minutes to see if you need to add more water.

When the vegetables are soft but not fully cooked add the rice and remove the lid. When the water has evaporated and the chicken is fully cooked, stir in the herbs and serve.

Cheat-Free Stir-fry

Servings: 6   **Cheats/Serving: 1**

If you don't have a leek, feel free to use an onion in this recipe. This can be combined with rice or quinoa.

1 tbsp coconut oil
2 garlic cloves, minced
1 leek, chopped
450g chicken or grass-fed beef, cut into strips
1 head broccoli, chopped into bite-size pieces
1 red pepper, sliced
400g sugar snap peas
200g tinned sliced water chestnuts, drained and rinsed
Fresh ginger, peeled and chopped, to taste
½ tbsp light soy sauce or tamari sauce

Add the olive oil to a wok and heat over a medium heat. When the oil is hot, add one garlic clove and the leek. When the leek is translucent, remove from the pan and set aside, leaving the oil in the pan.

Add the chicken or beef and the other garlic clove. Cook until the outside of the protein is done. Add the vegetables and stir-fry until they are cooked. (If there isn't enough oil, feel free to use water.) When the vegetables and protein are cooked, add in the leek, ginger and soy sauce. When leeks and ginger are heated through, remove and serve.

Chicken Marsala

Servings: 8   **Cheats/Serving: 2**

2 tbsp almond flour, divided
1 tsp minced garlic
1 tsp minced onions
1 tsp coarse sea salt
½ tsp coarsely ground black pepper
4 boneless, skinless, free-range chicken breasts, cut in
    half lengthwise
2 tbsp extra-virgin olive oil or coconut oil
200g mushrooms, sliced
125g chicken stock
175ml Marsala wine
1 tbsp butter
1 tsp basil leaves
Fresh parsley garnish

Add all but one tablespoon of the flour into a zip seal food storage bag. Add the garlic, onion, sea salt and ground black pepper, seal the bag and shake to mix.

Add the chicken breasts to the bag, re-seal, and shake to coat them thoroughly with the flour mixture.

Heat the olive oil in a large frying pan over medium-high heat,. When it's hot, cook several pieces of chicken three minutes per side, or until they are golden brown and no longer pink in the centre. Remove the chicken from the frying pan and keep it warm under a dish or foil. Repeat until all the chicken is cooked.

Add the mushrooms to the same frying pan and cook until tender, about five minutes.

Meanwhile, mix the stock and the reserved tablespoon of flour in a bowl. Add the mixture to the frying pan. Slowly stir in the wine. Bring this mixture to a boil, stirring to release the browned bits on the bottom of the frying pan.

Stir in the butter and add the basil, cooking for two more minutes, or until the sauce thickens.

Place the chicken on a serving dish, cover with the mushroom sauce and garnish with parsley flakes.

Chickpea and Spinach Curry with Cucumber-Avocado Sauce

Servings: 4   **Cheats/Serving: 1**

1 tbsp coconut oil
1 large onion, chopped
2 tbsp curry powder
4 garlic cloves, chopped
1 tbsp fresh ginger, chopped
500ml plus 1 tsp water
800g tinned chickpeas, drained and rinsed
600g spinach, chopped
1 cucumber, seeded and chopped
1 avocado, chopped
Juice of 1 lime
1 handful of coriander, chopped
Sea salt to taste
Large bowl of mixed greens
Lime wedges for garnish

Heat the oil in a large saucepan over a medium heat. Add the onion and fry until very light brown. Be sure to watch the onion so it doesn't burn.

Add the curry powder, garlic, ginger and one teaspoon of water to the pan and cook for 30 seconds.

Add the chickpeas, spinach and two cups of water to the saucepan. Bring to a simmer and cook until the mixture is slightly thickened, about 10 minutes.

While the chickpea mixture is cooking, add the cucumber, avocado, lime juice, coriander, and sea salt in a blender and blend until smooth.

Serve the chickpea mixture on a bed of mixed greens, topped with the sauce. Add lime wedges for garnish.

Ginger Salmon with Bok Choy and Spinach

Servings: 4   **Cheats/Serving: 2**

1 tbsp olive or coconut oil
Sea salt
450g skinless salmon fillet, sliced into 4 equal pieces
60ml (plus 1 tsp) water
4 spring onions, thinly sliced
2 garlic cloves, chopped
1 tbsp ginger, chopped
450g spinach
450g baby bok choy, halved lengthwise
Juice of 1 lime
1 tsp coriander (optional)
Chilli flakes to taste (optional)

Heat half a tablespoon of the oil in a large frying pan over medium-high heat. Season the salmon with sea salt and then cook in the frying pan, approximately 4–5 minutes per side.

In a separate frying pan over medium-high heat, add the remaining oil and one teaspoon of water. Add the spring onions, garlic and ginger and stir continuously for 30 seconds.

Add the spinach, bok choy and 60ml of water. Stir continuously for 4–6 minutes, or until the vegetables are just cooked and still bright green.

Place the salmon and vegetables on a plate and squeeze the lime juice over the top. Garnish with coriander and chilli flakes, if desired.

Grilled Lemon and Tamari Shrimp with Basil

Servings: 5   **Cheats/Serving: 3**

2 lemons, juiced
2 tbsp tamari or light soy sauce
4 tsp seafood seasoning
2 tsp ground black pepper
1 tsp dried basil
4 garlic cloves, minced
100ml olive oil
450g raw king prawns, peeled

Add all the ingredients except the king prawns to a large, zip seal food storage bag. Mix well and then add the prawns, making sure they are entirely covered. Refrigerate the prawns for at least 30 minutes.

Preheat the oven to 200°C/400°F/Gas Mark 6, or heat the grill to medium heat.

Cut a piece of foil large enough that all the shrimp will lay on top. Place the shrimp on the foil. Cut a second piece of foil the same size and place it over the top of the shrimp, crimping all the edges together. Make a slit in the top and then cook in the oven or under the grill for six minutes.

Honey Ginger Dijon Marinated Chicken Breasts

Servings: 8 to 12   **Cheats/Serving: 2**

100ml tamari or light soy sauce
125ml pineapple juice
60ml extra virgin olive oil
1 tsp Dijon mustard
1 tbsp honey
1 tsp ground ginger
1 tsp garlic
½ tsp freshly ground black pepper
1–6 boneless, skinless, free-range chicken breasts

Combine all the ingredients except the chicken in a large zip seal food storage bag and mix well. Add the chicken to the bag and refrigerate for 24 hours.

Grill the chicken until it is no longer pink in the centre.

Mussels with Coconut Curry Sauce

Servings: 14   **Cheats/Serving: 2**

This is the best coconut curry sauce recipe out there for mussels. There are subtle differences in this recipe that make it better than anything you'll see on the internet or even in gourmet restaurants. We make this claim after eating Sukanya Wicks recipe and also trying a disappointing version at a well-respected Colorado restaurant.

This sauce can also be used for almost any seafood. It also makes an excellent replacement for butter (try it with lobster!). You can also cook prawns, scallops, cod, halibut and even salmon using this recipe. Unlike the other recipes in this section, this one needs to be followed as closely as possible to achieve the precise flavour.

A hint here is that the combination of coriander, lime and spring onions will make or break this recipe. You want to make sure you have enough of this combination to bring out the flavour, but you don't want any single ingredient to overpower the others.

This is a great general rule of thumb when cooking with spices. Many people who are new to using spices tend to overdo it. While that is fine when you start, know that balance is the goal and this is what separates average cooks from great ones.

2kg mussels (preferably cultivated), scrubbed and rinsed
A little extra virgin olive oil
3 garlic cloves, minced
1 tbsp minced ginger (or more to taste)
½ tbsp Thai red curry paste (or more to taste)
½ small glass of dry white wine (optional)
1 tbsp sugar
400g coconut milk
1 large handful of coriander
About 3 spring onions, thinly sliced
Juice of 3 limes
1 tbsp slivered ginger
Lime wedges for garnish

Discard any mussels that are open and do not close when tapped (these are dead and will make you sick if you eat them). Scrub the mussels well and remove the beards. Cultivated mussels just need a good rinse.

Heat a pan over a medium-low heat. Add a tiny amount of olive oil and then sauté garlic and ginger for about 10 seconds. Add the curry paste, white wine, sugar and coconut milk. Cook over a high heat for about two minutes.

Add the mussels and coriander (saving some coriander for garnish) and toss well. Cover and cook the for 5–8 minutes.

Shake the pot a few times and discard any unopened mussels Garnish with more coriander, spring onions, lime juice and slivered ginger. Serve with lime wedges.

King Prawn Taco Wraps with Black Beans

Servings: 4   **Cheats/Serving: 1.5**

Swap the prawns for chicken for a variation on this recipe. The chicken should be seasoned with sea salt and cooked through, about 6–7 minutes on each side in a frying pan over a medium heat.

---

1 tbsp extra virgin olive oil
450g raw king prawns
Sea salt to taste
4 spring onions, sliced, white and green parts separated
800g tinned black beans, drained and rinsed
60ml water
½ avocado
Salsa
Coriander, chopped
4 lime wedges
1 large head of white cabbage, leaves separated

Heat half a tablespoon of the extra virgin olive oil in a large frying pan over a medium heat. Season the prawns with a little sea salt and cook in the frying pan until they're opaque and pink or orange, usually 3–5 minutes on each side.

In a separate pan, heat the remaining olive oil over a medium heat. Add the white parts of the spring onions, stirring until soft, 1–2 minutes.

Add the beans, water and a shake of sea salt. Cook until warmed through, about four minutes. Stir in the green parts of the spring onions.

To serve, place the bean mixture, prawns, chopped avocado, salsa, coriander and lime wedges into small bowls. Place the cabbage leaves on the table as wraps, and everyone can make their own.

Spicy Thai Curry

Servings: 8   **Cheats/Serving: 1 (2 per 1/2 cup rice)**

This curry is a gift that keeps on giving – make a huge pot and eat it over the next three days. It tastes better every time you reheat!

Curry is extremely customisable. Add whatever vegetables you like or have on hand and while I like basmati rice, brown rice is also good on the side.

1 aubergine
1 red pepper
1 yellow pepper
1 head broccoli
1 big carrot
400g coconut milk
2 tsp hot red or green Thai curry paste, or more to taste
2.5cm piece of ginger, minced
3 garlic cloves, minced
2 tbsp Thai basil, chopped
2 tbsp coriander, chopped
Basmati rice for serving

Chop the aubergine, peppers, broccoli and carrot into bite-sized pieces.

In a wok over medium-high heat, add the coconut milk, and then thoroughly incorporate the curry paste. When the coconut milk starts to simmer, add the vegetables. Add the ginger, garlic, Thai basil and coriander. Cook until the vegetables are done.

Sweet Orange and Paprika Chicken

Servings: 8 to 12   **Cheats/Serving: 1.5**

125ml freshly squeezed orange juice
½ tsp sea salt
¼ onion, minced
3 garlic cloves, minced
⅛ tsp paprika
⅛ tsp ground black pepper
4–6 boneless, skinless, free-range chicken breasts

Mix all the ingredients except the chicken in a zip seal food storage bag. Add the chicken and mix to coat the chicken completely. Place the bag in the refrigerator overnight, turning occasionally.

Remove the chicken from the bag, discarding the remaining marinade. Grill under a medium heat until tender, about 10 minutes.

Sauces

Orange Ginger Sauce for Stir-fry Fish or Chicken

Servings: 2   **Cheats/Serving: 1**

This is a great sauce for stir-fry. Either add it to your stir-fry at the end of cooking or gently heat it in a saucepan until it turns translucent, about five minutes.

3 oranges (add extra orange for more sauce)
1 tbsp vinegar
1 garlic clove (optional)
2.5cm ginger (optional)
2 tbsp tamari or light soy sauce
1 tsp sea salt

Remove the zest from two of the oranges.

In a bowl, add the juice of the oranges and the vinegar. Mince the garlic and ginger, if desired, and add to the bowl.

While whisking, add the tamari and sea salt

Peruvian Green Sauce

Servings: 2   **Cheats/Serving: 1**

Serve this on chicken, fish or pork. It's also great as a topper on any kind of cooked eggs. I love it on cooked string beans as well.

Add between one and three jalapeños, depending on how spicy you like things.

2 large handfuls of coriander, stems and all
1–3 jalapeños or green chillies, seeds removed
1 large garlic clove
½ tsp sea salt
2 tbsp extra virgin olive oil
2 tbsp water
1 tbsp lemon juice

Add ingredients to a food processor and process until smooth

High Nutrient Eats (With a Little Cheat on Top)

Brussels Sprouts with Bacon

Servings: 4   Cheats/Serving: 1

450g Brussels sprouts
1 tbsp extra virgin olive oil
3 bacon rashers, cooked

Bring a saucepan of water to boil (you only need enough water to cover the sprouts). Add the sprouts and boil for 10 minutes.

Drain the Brussels sprouts. When they're just cool enough to handle, cut each one in half.

Heat a pan over a medium heat. Add the olive oil. When the oil is hot, sauté the Brussels sprouts until golden brown. Crumble in the bacon and heat through.

Cauliflower Rice

Servings: 2   Cheats/Serving: 1

1 head of cauliflower
2 tbsp of coconut oil

Cut or blitz the cauliflower until it is the size of rice (use a food processor, grater or knife). Heat a frying pan on a medium-high heat. Add the oil when hot. Sauté the cauliflower with any seasonings desired (i.e. sea salt, garlic, ginger, curry, ground black pepper etc.). Stir frequently for 4 –5 minutes. Serve hot!

Cauliflower with Sweet Onion and Bacon

Servings: 2   Cheats/Serving: 1

Inspired by Cookfresh.

This yummy, nutrient dense, detoxifying powerhouse of a recipe that will fill you up and make you feel great. What I like about this it is that it uses just one herb in addition to sea salt and ground black pepper, making it really easy.

If you're craving warm mashed potatoes with bacon, try mashing the cauliflower. It has the same consistency as mashed potatoes!

2 bacon rashers (feel free to rock your inner bacon if need be)
3 garlic cloves, minced
1 onion, thinly sliced into 5cm strips
450g chopped cauliflower (usually a large head, chopped into 5cm pieces)
3 tbsp chicken stock
1 tsp rosemary, finely chopped
225g fresh spinach leaves
½ lemon, juiced
Sea salt and fresh ground black pepper to taste
1 tsp goat's cheese (optional)

In a large frying pan, cook the bacon over a medium-low heat until crisp. Use tongs to take out the bacon and place on a doubled paper towel. Drain most of bacon grease from the pan into a bowl, leave just a bit to cook the rest of the ingredients.

Over a medium heat, add the garlic, onion and cauliflower into the frying pan and stir until the cauliflower and onion start to turn a golden brown.

Add two tablespoons of chicken stock, the rosemary, and the spinach leaves, and cook until the cauliflower and spinach are tender, anywhere from 5–10 minutes. Remove from heat. Stir in the bacon, squeeze in the fresh lemon juice, and add sea salt and ground black pepper to desired taste. Add a teaspoon of crumbled goat's cheese on top if want.

Garlicky Mashed "Potatoes"

Servings: 2   **Cheats/Serving: 1**

Use butter infused with garlic and spices for an extra flavour in this recipe.

1 large head of cauliflower
5 garlic cloves
2 tbsp butter
Sea salt and ground black pepper to taste

Bring about 5cm of water to a boil in a stockpot. If you have a steamer insert, have it ready.

Wash and trim the cauliflower, and place it in the steamer (if you're using one) or add it directly to the stockpot. Cover and cook until the cauliflower is soft, about 10 minutes.

Drain the cauliflower very well using a colander. If you don't, your "potatoes" will be watery.

Place the cauliflower into a food processor or blender, then add the garlic and butter. Process until the cauliflower is smooth. Add sea salt and ground black pepper.

Perfect Sweet Potato Fries

Servings: 4   Cheats/Serving: 1

4 sweet potatoes
4 tbsp of extra virgin olive oil
Sea salt and ground black pepper to taste
Chilli flakes to taste

Preheat the oven to 230°C/450°F/Gas Mark 8.

Cut the sweet potatoes in half, keeping the skins on. Cut each half into large slices about 2cm thick, and cut those slices into fries 1–2cm wide.

Put the fries on a baking sheet, drizzle with olive oil, sea salt, ground black pepper and chilli flakes and mix with your hands, completely covering the sweet potato fries.

Flatten out the fries, so they aren't touching too much and bake in the oven for 15 minutes; after that period, flip and cook for 10 more minutes. You might need less time if you like them less done, or more time if you like them super crispy.

Roasted Broccoli or Asparagus

Servings: 3   Cheats/Serving: 1

1kg vegetables: broccoli, asparagus, cauliflower, carrots, courgette, onion, mushrooms, green beans, beets, swede, turnips, peppers, whatever your fancy!
3 tbsp extra virgin olive oil
1 tsp sea salt

Preheat the oven to 180°C/350°F/Gas Mark 4. Cut all the vegetables into similar sized pieces. In a large bowl, add the vegetables and oil, and mix well with your hands. Add the sea salt and mix again.

Spread the vegetables evenly on a baking tray or casserole dish (aim for a single layer) and roast for 10 minutes for wet vegetables and 20 to 30 minutes for dense vegetables.

Simple Sautéed Spinach

Servings: 2   **Cheats/Serving: 0**

If your children don't care for spinach, serve mustard or soy sauce on the side for dipping. This trick works great for green beans, too. If you want to add a little more flavour, chop up a couple of garlic cloves and fry them in the olive oil before adding the spinach.

If you don't have fresh spinach, there is nothing wrong with frozen. Frozen spinach is also cheaper. Overall, spinach is inexpensive and can be very tasty if made right.

2 tsp extra virgin olive oil
450g fresh or frozen spinach
Chilli flakes to taste
Sea salt to taste

Heat a saucepan over a medium-high. When it's hot add the olive oil then add the spinach.

Use a wooden spoon or spatula to stir the spinach for about three minutes. Add the chilli flakes and sea salt and stir for one minute. Serve hot.

Sweet Potatoes

Servings: 4   Cheats/Serving: 0

4 sweet potatoes
1 large onion, diced
½ tsp sea salt
¼ tsp ground black pepper

Preheat the oven to 200°C/400°F/Gas Mark 6.

Pierce the potatoes a few times with a fork and place them on a baking sheet. Bake for 45 minutes, until they're tender. Meanwhile, heat the oil in a frying pan over a medium heat. Once it's hot, sauté the onion for 10–15 minutes, until it's caramelised. Once the potatoes are done, cut a slit on the top and add the caramelized onion, sea salt and ground black pepper.

Sweet Potatoes Bacon Bakes

Servings: 4   Cheats/Serving: 4

4 tbsp extra virgin olive oil
8 bacon rashers
4 large garlic cloves, minced
½ tsp sea salt
½ tsp ground black pepper
4 medium sweet potatoes
50g toasted flaked almonds

Preheat the oven to 220°C/425°F/Gas Mark 6.

Heat a tablespoon of the oil in a frying pan over a medium heat. Add the bacon and cook for 10 minutes.

Meanwhile, in a mixing bowl, combine the remaining oil, garlic, sea salt and ground black pepper.

Cut pieces of foil into four pieces large enough to wrap each potato loosely.

Rub each potato with the oil mixture, and then wrap each potato in foil and seal by pinching the ends together.

Bake the potatoes on a baking sheet for 40 minutes. Garnish with the bacon and almonds.

Apps, Desserts and Extras

Appetizers

Amazing Tart Lime Mango Salsa

Servings: 6   **Cheats/Serving: 1**

My mother-in-law first served a version of this with tangerine on an unusually warm July day in Maine, and as I watched her slave over the tangerine preparation, I thought, wouldn't it be so much easier with mango?

The very next day we substituted the mango and voilà! My favourite salsa was born. The mix of the tart lime and the sweet mango are to die for.

This can be used as a topping to tilapia, salmon or grilled chicken, and it's fantastic on top of a piping-hot bowl of black beans. It's even a great way to cool down a soup or add a boost of flavour to sweet potatoes or squash. I prefer it at room temperature.

Here's the best secret of all: this salsa helps make bad food taste good! If you're invited to a barbecue or dinner, it's a great dish to bring because if you don't care for the fare, you'll have a wonderful topping to mask the mediocre food.

It's a great recipe to keep in the fridge because you can make a large bowl of it and munch all day. With vitamins C and A, mango, and cleansing little cucumber bites, it's a great nutrient addition to any meal.

3 mangos
1 large cucumber
¼ red onion, finely chopped
1 handful coriander, chopped, a bit reserved for garnish
¼ jalapeño or green chilli, finely chopped
Juice of 1 lime (or more to taste)

Peel the mango and slice into 2.5cm cubes. Peel the cucumber and cut lengthwise. Scoop out the seeds with a spoon and discard. Dice cucumber into 2.5cm cubes. Place in a large bowl. Add coriander, jalapeño and lime juice. Sprinkle a bit of the coriander on top and add a lime wedge for presentation, if desired.

Beef, Chilli Beans and Salsa Mexican Dip

Servings: 6   **Cheats/Serving: 1**

450g grass-fed beef
500g salsa
400g tinned chilli beans, drained and rinsed
50g tinned sliced olives
3 spring onions, sliced
2 tomatoes, chopped

Preheat the oven to 180°C/350°F/Gas Mark 4. In a frying pan over medium-high heat, cook the minced beef thoroughly. Stir in the salsa, then reduce the heat and simmer for 20 minutes, or until the liquid is absorbed.

Stir in the beans and cook until they're thoroughly heated. Place the mixture in a bowl and sprinkle the olives, spring onion and tomatoes on top.

Joanie's Artichoke Tapenade

Servings: 4   **Cheats/Serving: 1**

2 garlic cloves
1 handful raw spinach
¼ tsp sea salt
¼ onion, sliced
1 tsp ground black pepper
1 tbsp extra virgin olive oil
1 tbsp tahini
50g olives (optional)
400g tinned artichoke hearts, drained
1 large tomato, chopped
2 tbsp pine nuts
1 handful coriander (optional)

Add the garlic, spinach, sea salt, onion, ground black pepper, olive oil, tahini and olives to a food processor and process until it's smooth. Add the artichoke hearts, tomato, pine nuts and coriander and pulse until slightly chunky. Serve immediately.

Spicy Ranch Dressing with Baked Chicken Wings

Ranch Dressing Servings: 4   **Cheats/Serving: 1**
Chicken Wings Servings: 2   **Cheats/Serving: 5**

This ranch dressing recipe is great because you don't have to have any fresh ingredients – you can just use dried spices and still have your favourite ranch (but without preservatives). It's best paired with grilled barbecue chicken on top of 450g of mixed greens.

Spicy Ranch Dressing
4 tbsp Hellmann's mayo (it must be Hellmann's!)
3 tbsp apple cider vinegar

¼ tsp dried dill weed or herbs de Provence
⅛ tsp dried basil
¼ tsp dried garlic
¼ tsp granulated onion
¼ to tsp cayenne pepper
⅛ tsp sea salt
⅛ tsp ground black pepper

Chicken Wings
3 tbsp extra virgin olive oil
2 garlic cloves, minced
2 tsp chilli powder
1 tsp garlic powder
Sea salt and ground black pepper to taste
10 chicken wings

Preheat the oven to 190°C/375°F/Gas Mark 5.

First make the dressing. In a food processor, process the mayo and apple cider vinegar to incorporate. Add the rest of the ingredients and blend well.

Now for the chicken wings. Combine the olive oil, garlic, chilli powder, garlic powder, sea salt and ground black pepper in a zip seal food storage bag. Seal the bag and shake to combine the ingredients.

Add the chicken wings to the bag, reseal, and shake well to coat. Arrange the chicken wings on a baking sheet.

Cook for one hour, until crisp and cooked through (no longer dark pink in the middle).

Perfect Mexican Guacamole

Servings: 6   **Cheats/Serving: 1**

This guacamole is great served with thin slices of cucumber or oven-baked chicken.

2 ripe avocados
1 tbsp freshly squeezed lime juice
½ tsp sea salt
2 spring onions, sliced
1 handful coriander, finely chopped
2 tbsp light or home-made mayonnaise (optional)
1 tomato, diced

Halve the avocados, scoop the flesh into a bowl, and discard the pit. Add the lime juice.

Mash well with a fork or potato masher, and then add the sea salt, onions, coriander and mayonnaise. Once everything is mixed well, fold in the tomatoes.

Pico de Gallo

Servings: 8   **Cheats/Serving: 0**

This piquant sauce from Mexico means beak of a rooster. Traditionally a dip for tortillas, it's a breeze to prepare. Add it to your avocado, quesadillas, black beans, eggs, grilled fish, tuna fish, hamburgers, or like some aficionados I know, just eat it right out of the bowl. I dip my toasted poppadoms into this salsa. You can also substitute two ripe mangos for the tomatoes.

6 tomatoes, chopped
1 small red onion, chopped
1 handful coriander, chopped (or more to taste)
1 jalapeño or green chilli pepper (or more to taste)

Juice of 1 lime
¼ tsp lime zest
Sea salt to taste

Place all the ingredients in a bowl and mix well.

King Prawn and Lime Appetiser with Parsley

Servings: 2   **Cheats/Serving: 1**

2 handfuls mixed greens
16 cooked king prawns
Juice of 1 lime
8 tbsp flat-leaf parsley, chopped

Place the greens on an serving plate and then arrange the prawns. Squeeze the entire lime over the platter, and then sprinkle the fresh parsley over the top.

Spring Fresh Cherry Tomato Appetiser

Servings: 4   **Cheats/Serving: 1**

This is a great addition to any traditional protein, such as grilled chicken, or on top of a bed of mixed greens.

225g cherry tomatoes
6 garlic cloves
1 handful coriander, chopped
100g artichoke hearts, quartered and rinsed
4 tbsp extra virgin olive oil
Juice of ½ lemon
1–2 tsp dried red chilli flakes (or more to taste)
Sea salt and ground black pepper to taste
Goat's cheese

Halve the cherry tomatoes. Grind the garlic cloves. Chop the coriander leaves, tossing the stems.

Put the chopped ingredients in a large mixing bowl with the artichoke hearts and mix.

Add the lemon juice, red chilli flakes, sea salt and ground black pepper and mix everything well.

Top with a little crumbled goat's cheese, if desired.

Toasted Rosemary Almonds

Servings: 6   **Cheats/Serving: 1.5**

1½ cups flaked almonds
½ tsp rosemary, chopped
⅛ tsp sea salt

Place a large frying pan over a medium heat. Add the almonds to the frying pan and heat until they turn a light golden colour and you can start to smell the almond oils, 7–10 minutes. Gently stir to allow for even toasting.

Remove from the pan and place in bowl, stirring in rosemary and sea salt.

Desserts

Cinna-Raisin Cookies

Servings: 6   Cheats/Serving: 1

These cookies make a great after-school treat!

50g almond flour or ground almonds
3 tbsp ground walnuts
1 tbsp ground cinnamon
⅛ tsp allspice
⅛ tsp nutmeg
1 tbsp honey
2 tbsp currants
50g raisins
1 omega-3 enriched egg

Preheat the oven to 180°C/350°F/Gas Mark 4.

In a large bowl, mix together the flour, walnuts, cinnamon, allspice and nutmeg. Add the honey, currants, raisins and egg and mix well.

Form small balls and place them on a oven tray. Bake for 20–30 minutes.

Cinnamon Candied Walnuts

Servings: 4   Cheats/Serving: 2.5

25g granulated sugar
175g raw walnut halves
Pinch of sea salt
2 tsp ground cinnamon

Preheat the oven to 180°C/350°F/Gas Mark 4.

Lay the walnuts out on a baking sheet in a single layer. Bake for five minutes. They could need one or two more minutes; just be careful not to burn them. Make sure you stay in the kitchen to keep your eye on them! After they are toasted, remove them from the oven and allow them to cool.

Pour the sugar into a medium saucepan. Cook the sugar on medium heat, stirring with a wooden spoon as soon as the sugar begins to melt. Keep stirring until all the sugar has melted and it changes to a medium-amber to medium-caramel colour. Immediately add the walnuts to the pan, quickly stirring and coating each piece.

As soon as the walnuts are coated with the sugar, spread them out on a rimmed baking sheet, lined with parchment paper. Use tongs or forks (don't use your fingers the sugar is extremely hot!) to separate the walnuts from each other, working very quickly. Sprinkle the nuts with the sea salt and cinnamon.

Easiest Apple Cinnamon Dessert

Servings: 2   **Cheats/Serving: 1**

2 apples, peeled, cored and chopped
1 tsp raw sugar
1 tsp cinnamon

In a small, microwave-safe bowl, mix the apple, sugar and cinnamon. Microwave for one minute on high.

Fantastic Banana Bread

Servings: 12   **Cheats/Serving: 3**

Banana bread on a diet? Yes! This recipe is my mom's. When I realised it had three Cheats a slice, I wanted to see if I could cheatify it. Every recipe I found online either had tons of sugar and fat (one recipe I found had raisins, orange juice, and nuts!) or was so chock full of chemicals (another recipe had a ½ cup of equal sugar substitute!) that I couldn't recommend anything else.

If you love banana bread, this recipe is great. It has all natural ingredients and is well worth "spending" three Cheats on!

250g plain white flour
1 tsp baking soda
¼ tsp sea salt
100g butter
170g dark brown sugar
2 eggs, beaten
500g ripe bananas (about 4 medium), mashed
120g walnuts and pecans (or walnuts and chocolate chips)

Preheat the oven to 180°C/350°F/Gas Mark 4. Lightly grease a 22-by-12cm loaf tin.

In a large bowl, combine the flour, baking soda and sea salt. In separate bowl, cream together the butter and dark brown sugar. Stir in the eggs and mashed bananas until well blended.

Stir the banana mixture into the flour mixture just enough to moisten everything. Add the nuts and just incorporate them. Pour the batter into the prepared loaf tin.

Bake 60–65 minutes, until a skewer inserted into the centre of the loaf comes out clean. Allow the loaf cool in the pan for 10 minutes, and then let it finish cooling on a wire rack.

Gajar Halwa

Servings: 8   **Cheats/Serving: 1**

This is a low-fat version of a divine dessert fit for an emperor. Traditionally, it's oozing in ghee and exceedingly sweet. In India, it's served covered with edible silver leaf.

The halwa can be eaten warm or at room temperature.

---

2 tbsp ghee
1 tbsp flaked almonds
1 tbsp unroasted and unsalted pistachios
4 green cardamom pods
4 medium carrots, grated
6 tbsp low-fat ricotta
70g brown sugar
2 tbsp golden raisins
Rosewater for sprinkling

Heat the ghee in a heavy-bottomed pan over a medium heat. When heated, fry the almonds and pistachios. Remove the nuts and set aside.

Add the cardamom and lightly sauté for two minutes.

Add the grated carrots and sauté for 10 minutes or until the liquid is absorbed, stirring frequently so as not to burn.

Add the ricotta, brown sugar, and raisins. Cook the mixture over a low heat until the ghee pulls away, about 15 minutes.

Remove to a serving dish. Sprinkle with the almonds and pistachios on top and just before serving sprinkle with rosewater.

Pumpkin Pie

Servings: 2   **Cheats/Serving: 1**

This recipe can help satiate your sweet tooth as well as give you and your family a huge dose of vitamin A, a critical nutrient in keeping the immune system strong. This can literally be made in a matter of minutes. While lacking the exact flavour and structure of pumpkin pie, if you love pumpkin, this can be a great thing to whip up at the last minute.

Also, kids love this. (We have proven this through clinical research.)

400g tinned puréed pumpkin
½ tbsp coconut oil or butter
3 tbsp sugar or 1 tbsp molasses (optional)
1 tsp cinnamon
⅛ tsp ground ginger (optional)
⅛ tsp nutmeg (optional)
Pinch of sea salt

Put the puréed pumpkin in a microwave-safe bowl. Add the coconut oil and mix. Add the sugar, cinnamon, ginger, nutmeg and sea salt.

Microwave for three minutes. Remove, stir and cool. Add or adjust the flavours as you like.

Raspberry Parfait

Servings: 2   **Cheats/Serving: 2**

400g low-fat Greek yogurt
200g raspberries
1 tbsp honey
2 tsp flaked almonds

Put yogurt in a small bowl, and then top with the other ingredients.

Rj Pops

Servings: 4   **Cheats/Serving: 1**

This recipe calls for ice lolly moulds. These pops are a fun, refreshing treat on a warm day.

150g fresh or frozen raspberries
150g coconut milk
1 medium banana
½ lemon, juiced
1 tbsp honey
1 egg white

In a blender, blend the raspberries, milk, banana, lemon juice and honey until creamy.

In a mixing bowl, whisk the egg white with a hand mixer until soft peaks have formed.

Gently fold the raspberry mixture into egg whites. Pour the mixture into the lolly moulds and freeze.

Spiced Summer Fruit Compote

Servings: 8   Cheats/Serving: 1

Let your slow cooker cook this light, healthy dessert while you spend the day on the beach or reading in your hammock. Alternatively, you can poach the peaches in a non-reactive saucepan for 30 minutes, or until tender.

250ml white wine, apple or pineapple juice
4 tbsp honey
¼ lemon, thinly sliced
2.5cm piece of ginger, julienned
3 cardamom pods
3 cloves
8 ripe but firm peaches, halved and stones removed
600g berries of your choice
Rosewater for sprinkling
Fresh mint leaves for garnish

In a saucepan, heat the wine, honey, lemon, ginger, cardamom and cloves until bubbling. Add the peaches and spoon the syrup over the top. Cover and cook over low heat for 90 minutes.

Remove the cardamom, cloves, and lemon slices. Place the peaches in a serving bowl, pour the sauce over the top and gently mix in the berries. Sprinkle with rosewater and garnish with mint leaves.

Watermelon Sorbet

Servings: 2   **Cheats/Serving: 1**

Watermelon is an interesting fruit. It is relatively low in calories for a fruit, with roughly 40–50 calories per one-cup serving. There are between 75–100 calories in the average slice of watermelon.

Watermelons have a fairly good calorie-to-nutrient ratio. They are rich in vitamin A and C (like most fruit) and also contain some B vitamins, which are thought to be good for energy.

Watermelons also score well on Dr. Fuhrman's system that factors how many nutrients there are per calorie. Watermelons are rich in a substance called lycopene, which has been shown to be a powerful antioxidant. This sorbet has no added sugar. It's easy and very inexpensive to make.

600g watermelon flesh, cut into chunks
Juice of 1 lime
1 handful raspberries
1 mint sprig for garnish

Freeze the watermelon overnight.

Place the frozen watermelon in a blender and purée until smooth. If you like your sorbet sour, add the lime juice.

Serve topped with raspberries and garnished with mint.

Drinks

Muscle Recovery Margaritas

Servings: 8   Cheats/Serving: 2

This recipe makes enough for a small party. I suggest making the recipe in two stages as the party progresses.

1 bottle tequila
1kg frozen blueberries
Small amount of fresh ginger (careful – a little goes a long way!)
2 handfuls of fresh mint
6–8 limes
Ice

In a blender, mix half a bottle of tequila with a bag of frozen blueberries. Add a 2.5cm piece of ginger, the fresh mint and the juice of 3–4 limes.

Blend until you reach the desired consistency, adding ice to dilute the recipe as needed. Repeat these steps upon making the second batch.

Nearly Cheat-Free Hot Chocolate

Servings: 2   Cheats/Serving: 0.5

500ml unsweetened coconut milk
2 tbsp cocoa

Combine the ingredients in a small saucepan. Heat on a low heat until warm.

Virgin Piña Colada

Servings: 2   **Cheats/Serving: 1**

500ml unsweetened coconut milk
250g frozen pineapple

Add all the ingredients to a blender and blend until smooth.

Warm Chocolove Hot Chocolate

Servings: 2   **Cheats/Serving: 1**

If you need warm emotional goodness at night, try this recipe inspired by the Chocolove Almonds and Sea salt in Dark Chocolate bar.

500ml almond milk
1 tbsp almond butter
2 medjool dates, de-stoned
2 tbsp cocoa powder
2 tsp hemp seeds (optional)

Add all the ingredients to a blender and blend on high until smooth. Place the mixture in saucepan and heat until piping hot. You can also microwave it in a microwave-safe container until hot.

CHAPTER 10

The Cheats and Eats Lifestyle Programme Maintenance Plan

How to Keep the Weight You've Lost Off – For Good

One of the most important ways to manifest integrity is to be loyal to those who are not present.

— STEPHEN COVEY

You're probably expecting to hear another "plan" in this chapter, including how many Cheats you get to eat and how much exercise you have to do. We'll definitely talk about that but first I want to discuss the most important part of the maintenance plan: how you're going to keep the weight off long term.

You've just spent three weeks changing your life. You've been making positive changes for yourself or maybe even your family, too, and the people around you have noticed. Your friends, who questioned why you were ordering a huge and delicious salad instead of the risotto at dinner, start to ask you what you've done to look so great; the co-worker who swears by her tough-as-nails, 90-minute spin class but still has a belly demands to know what exercise class you took to get rid of yours.

Or maybe you're just on your way there. Maybe you've lost some weight and aren't at your goal weight yet, but you are enjoying how you feel on The Cheats and Eats Lifestyle Programme. Or maybe you slipped up a little too often and know that you could do better.

Wherever you are, if you've done three weeks on The Cheats and Eats Lifestyle Programme you have succeeded in your goal to make this diet different.

Now is the time for you to figure out how you're going to Cheat and Eat for longer than just the three weeks. Even though all the people around you say that they want to know what you've done to look so great, in reality, those people will probably end up being the same people who question your good choices going forward. Sometimes your friends, family, co-workers – really anyone in your life – will question your choices because it brings up their own issues, which they haven't dealt with. Sometimes slights can really get to us. In those situations, how do you cope?

How Can You be Positive in a World That Naturally Leans Negative?

I overheard a conversation when I was in Aspen, Colorado, over the summer. Two women were clearly seeing each other for the first time in months. The minute they said "Hi," one complimented the other. "Wow, you look great!"

And the other woman responded, "Are you kidding? Why do I even pay my trainer? Look at the inside of my thighs!"

The other woman replied, "Your thighs? Look at my jiggly arm fat!"

That conversation is typical. I bet you've said something similar. We all do, because as a society, but especially as women, we tend to bond over what's wrong with us – what's wrong with our job, what's wrong with our body, our face, our hair – instead of what's actually going right and what's amazingly awesome about us. This negativity usually extends past ourselves to other people – it's delicious to exchange gossip, because we get useful information about others in our social circle that way – and getting that view into other people's lives and troubles makes us feel better about our own life.

Most people feel uncomfortable talking positively about their lives because society has put a total clampdown on talking about success.

Talking about your own development and your efforts to better yourself is definitely not considered "cool" and it's usually considered bragging by most people. You're never supposed to talk about what you're excited about, whether it's a job or the guy you're dating or your kids excelling in a class or a sport. We're stuck in a place where it's unacceptable to want to improve your life.

For this maintenance plan, I want you to find friends who really are supportive, who are comfortable with you being great. I have made this a must-have in my life and it's improved my daily life and health dramatically. Whenever I express anxiety or frustration, my friends will remind me of what I want – and how all of those negative things tend to fade away when I concentrate on what's going well in my life.

Don't Ride the Negative Spiral With Yourself or With Others – Focus On What's *Right*

For you to continue the path you're on – which is a positive, awesome, life-changing path – you need to make sure you get love and support from people who aren't riding the negative spiral downwards.

Just like you have moved away from the Cheats and toward the Eats on your plate, you can begin to tip the scales from the negative to the positive within yourself, your social circle and even your family members. You can start a shift of what you bond over with each of your friends and family members, even your spouse.

This can be tough to do, because our brains are hard-wired to focus on what's going wrong (because, remember, our brains see it as a problem to solve). It's important to remind yourself of what's *right*, what's *working*, what's *good* in your life. That helps you see a hurdle as what it is – an obstacle to get over, instead of a giant stop sign. You can start by trying to bond over the smallest positive things, which can be powerful. Start with one person. Learn how to avoid self-deprecation (and enabling it) by offering that one person help, advice and ideas instead of falling into the muck.

It might be difficult, especially if you have always connected with your best friend, or your spouse, or your parent about what's bad or not working in your life. But it's worth trying because once you find that person who will be positive and offer you support and love without bringing you down, it will give you so much joy and help you keep improving yourself.

This is all about well-being. This is not just about diet, it's about being a happier, healthier you. For more information on well-being and how to continue on that awesome life-changing path visit Healthspan's website (www.healthspan.co.uk).

This Is Your Year

Now is the time for you to focus on you. Specifically, how great you are. The advice in this chapter so far may sound woo-woo or hippie-dippie, but it's really not. (If you try it, you'll see how grounded it is.) When working with people that are trying to lose weight we've always challenged them to tackle their relationships and how they interact with the world at the same time they are tackling their weight, because all of these things are tied into your identity. And once you start to change one of these elements in your life, your identity begins to shift – and all the other pieces must shift as well in order to make the whole puzzle fall into place.

The Rest of the Puzzle

You may have noticed that you have more energy during the day, that you sleep better at night, that the bags under your eyes aren't there anymore, that you are in flow more often than not when you exercise. You've probably begun to know instinctively how you're going to Cheat and Eat throughout the day, perhaps even throughout your week. Maybe people have mentioned that you're smiling more, that you have become a positive force in their lives.

These are all ways you can tell that the work you are doing on The Cheats and Eats Lifestyle Programme is affecting how you feel long after the initial three-week period you've just been through. This plan is not all about your weight – it's about the problems that your weight was a symptom of. And in order to keep the weight you've lost off, it's important to be conscious of not only what you eat, how you exercise and what you weigh but also how you're feeling – so you can avoid slipping back to the place you were at when you started reading this book.

The rest of this chapter focuses on the nuts and bolts: how many Cheats you can have per day when you're in maintenance mode; how you should alter the exercise plan; how to figure out whether you're at the weight you should be, what to do if you suddenly see an increase in the number on the scale and how to be the best advocate for your own health for the rest of your life. However, like the rest of The Cheats and Eats Lifestyle Programme, these practical pieces don't make the maintenance puzzle complete without the emotional component. So be sure to monitor how you're feeling as much as you do the number on the scale.

Tipping the Scale

Earlier in the book, we mentioned that the Cheats and Eats should be seen as two sides of a scale. In maintenance mode, we want you to tip the scale even farther – as far as you can – to the Eats side.

Eating even more Eats will build up the level of micronutrients in your body so that it's easier for your body to recover if and when you mess up or choose to "binge" on Cheats. When you really focus on the Eats, three slices of pizza on Wednesday night with your kids won't automatically mean two more pounds on the scale.

Though you *can* go up to 10 Cheats per day once you're in maintenance mode, we encourage people to really focus on the Eats. Save your Cheats for the night you want to have fish and chips with your kids, or the evening out with your spouse or that special occasion.

Exercise: Build Upon Your Base

Now that you understand the concept of building your base, you can begin to go faster in your workouts and push yourself more. Just remember what Dr. Phil Maffetone says: Don't get hung up on time. If you've planned to work out for an hour one day, but 15 minutes in you're starting to stress out about the laundry, your to-do list, and you begin dreading the amount of time you're spending in the workout, stop right there. Personally, I can't even think of doing an hour-long yoga class because 20 minutes in, I always end up worrying about all the things I've got to do that day. But if I just do 20 minutes, it's bliss. Treat your workouts the same.

Also, the more you can change *how* you move – by incorporating different classes, exercises, sports and activities – the more you will build your complementary muscles and the better you will look and feel. Try a new sport – if you haven't already done so, try something you liked when you were younger or just something entirely new to you.

My mother went hang-gliding for the first time and said that it was the thrill of her life and gave her more confidence in her physical abilities. I recently bought the video game Just Dance so I could enjoy the movement I love with my daughter.

The important thing is that you keep doing what works for you. The Cheats and Eats Lifestyle Programme exercise plan doesn't change all that much in terms of *what* you should do (or for how long, because less is more when it comes to exercise), but how you're doing it. Now that you have a base of exercise you're comfortable with – and that doesn't stress your body out – and you have begun to restore your complementary muscles, your workouts should simply build upon that foundation.

Your "Perfect" Weight

This is not a myth. **Everyone has a perfect weight.** You can tell you're at the perfect weight when you have energy, feel good about yourself, and can try on a dress or a pair of jeans without worrying about how they'll fit. You look great in clothes, but your face doesn't look drawn (which can mean you're below your perfect weight).

You know you've reached equilibrium in mind and body when your weight is like a rubber band – it might go up a pound or two after a night out or a vacation, but it's not long before you're back at the right number.

There comes a time where you instinctively know what to eat in any situation, whether it's an office party, having dinner at your in-laws, or being in a hurry and grabbing something from the high-street to take to your meeting at work. It's like driving a car: when you first got behind the wheel, you checked your rear-view mirror, your side mirrors and double-checked that everything was right before turning the car on. Now, years later, all those things are automatic and easy for you without much thought. The Cheats and Eats Lifestyle Programme will be the same way.

"How often should I weigh myself?"

This is very important, since it helps monitor your progress, or confirm that you're a pound or two away from (remember the rubber band) or are at, your perfect weight. Do what works for you. Some people prefer to weigh themselves once a week, others every day. Use the scales as a way to monitor your weight but don't become a slave to them. You may also choose an item of clothing to focus on as your goal, maybe this is your favourite pair of jeans you have been trying to get into or a dress you have brought for a special occasion.

The Secret of People Who Keep It Off

According to US life coach, Tony Robbins, people who are successful at weight loss have a number in their head of where they want to be. When the number they see on the scale goes up by more than two or three pounds, it sets off an alarm in their head: *Danger! You are off track! Danger! Get Back on Track!* This is the number one habit of people who have been successful, long term, at maintaining their weight loss.

I hear what you're thinking: "Jackie, you're so focused on the scale. Shouldn't we be focused on health, because after all, I'm building muscle and muscle weighs more than fat... " And you definitely have a point. I have a neighbour who showed me a picture. She's five foot nine and 10 stone in both photos, but one was taken before she started building muscle and one was taken after. She saw the exact same number on the scale, but she looks drastically different in those photos. Her clothes fit differently, and her body looks transformed.

But here's the truth: whether you're "building muscle" or not, it's important to be comfortable with your *number*. Hitting that number has to make you feel confident in yourself and great overall. When you're not comfortable with your number – when you make it too low or even sometimes too high – you subtly sabotage yourself because you don't really think you can hit it or that it will make you feel awesome.

It can be easier to start with a range, or a number you want to be *below*. For some women, it's under 10 stone. Some it's under nine stone. For a lot of guys, it's being under 14 stone. Whatever it is, try to find your true number or range and stick to it. Keep your weight loss alarm bell set to ready, so that anytime you see a number that's two digits higher, it goes off.

What I see a lot, is that when people have succeeded for a while at losing weight, they forget how hard they've worked to get there. So, they slack off – or eat more Cheats than normal. Next thing they know, the number they are seeing is three, four, five, maybe even 10 pounds over their number – and those people start to hide. They turn down invitations, they start to miss out on the very things that make us all feel great – connection and fun with our friends.

But that won't happen to you if you keep focusing on the Eats and keep that alarm bell on ready. And don't press the snooze button. Make it really loud and when it goes off, get up.

Conclusion: Why You Can Lose Weight Now

Twenty years from now you will be more disappointed
by the things that you didn't do than by the ones you did do
— MARK TWAIN

You might be thinking, "Ok, but how am I actually going to do this. I understand it's a list. I eat as much as I want from the Eat side and I just count my Cheats. I stop burning myself out and beating myself up when I haven't gotten to the gym. And I can still eat my cheese and lose weight. But I've tried this before. I have every best intention to start on Monday and I get thrown off. Or I'm great all day and I mess up at night. Why is this going to be different? How can I really do it this time? Because I need to. I have to do this. I want to look good. I want to feel good. I want to be back where I know I'm in the zone and I'm getting it done."

I think this happens to almost everyone who reads a diet book. You read the entire thing, thinking the whole time "this all sounds great, but can I really do it?" You can. You will succeed on The Cheats and Eats Lifestyle Programme. Here's why:

1. Nothing is Off the Table

If you really love your coffee with sugar in the morning or having a glass of wine in the evening, you don't have to give that up. You simply just have to count it as a cheat. Nothing is ever off-limits, period.

The Cheats and Eats Lifestyle Programme is a list – with everything included. We've designed the system so that we do the work for you. You eat your Eats and limit your Cheats with a few exceptions to the rules. Your focus on eats will negate the body blows of the cheats and this will become so automatic, you won't even think about it. You aren't focused on fibre, or fat or nutrients. We've done that for you. You eat your Eats, and you limit your Cheats.

2.There's No Such Thing as Failure

If you sat on the couch all week, you can still succeed on this diet. If you binged on crisps last night, you can still succeed on this diet. Whatever you feel like you did that was "bad" or "wrong" can be overcome on this diet.

When you accept that you can't fail, no matter what, you will be able to shift your focus from what you are unable to do or are doing "wrong" to what's possible, doable and going right. When you shift your focus, it's far easier to follow through and succeed.

You don't have to beat yourself up anymore that you haven't embraced the latest churn and burn craze. You don't have to feel bad that you ate a piece of bread. You will feel good about your small successes and they will lead to you losing the weight.

3. The Weekly One Thing

The "weekly one thing" is a great solution for people who have no idea where to start. The thought of starting anywhere seems too overwhelming. If you're thinking, "How can I do this? I have three kids, I've done this before, everything I try doesn't work, I'm great all day but then I mess up at night, I am in so much trouble at work, maybe I can start this in three weeks…". Then this is the solution for you.

When you're in the middle of living your life, figuring out where to start can be really tough. That's why we asked you, at the beginning of the book, to pick just one thing that's tripping you up. Did you pick that one thing and focus on changing it? If so, what was it? Were you successful? How did that make you feel? Can you pick one more thing that you want to start changing?

Whether you participated in that "one thing" exercise at the beginning or not, now is the time for you to pick something. If you're not sure where to start, simply focus on one thing that's tripping you up – and focus on changing that one thing. It can be anything: late night snacking, avoiding doughnuts at the office, not buying crisps, whatever. You don't have to fix everything all at once; you can start just by picking one thing.

When you put your energy and your focus into changing this one thing, you will change how you feel. And if you turn the one thing into a "weekly one thing" – changing one thing a week about your diet or lifestyle – you will slowly build momentum and transition into a mode that, because I don't know how else to describe it, is hopeful. I actually call it "hope mode" with the people I talk too. Being in hope mode is so powerful; it will make every challenge seem conquerable and make you feel undefeatable. And it all starts with just one thing.

4. You Can Do This and You Will Do This – Because This Is *Your* Year

What do I mean by that? I mean that *this* is the year you're going to make a change. *This is the year you will succeed.* Write "this is the year" on a piece of paper and tape it to your mirror; put it in your phone as an alarm. Remind yourself of it like a mantra: *this is the year. This is the year. This is the year. This is* **my** *year.*

That's the truth. *It is* **your** *year*. What you've done in the past – the failures, the successes, everything that could have been – it has all built to this coming year, when things will be different. This is the year when things will change. You might be reading this in November, or May, or August. It doesn't matter because the next 365 days is all about you. Those next 365 days is when your life, your weight and your happiness will change. Because The Cheats and Eats Lifestyle Programme will give you momentum that you haven't had before, the momentum you need to make this *your* year.

This is not the year to *think* about this being the year, what you're going to do or what you want to do from your life; this is the year to *do* everything you've wanted. This is your year – and I promise you that once you begin to take that on, you will experience flow and fly. You will experience more daily success than you have before, and build the momentum and push to accomplish all the goals you want to over the next year.

Believing that this is your year helps you live in the mode of hope. It gets you in your zone. When you're in the zone, "bang-ups and hang-ups still happen to you" but you quickly remind yourself, this is the year. You get that feeling, that special knowing feeling that things are going to be different this time.

This is the year when you make the change. This is your year to be successful by focusing on the Eats and choosing your Cheats. It's just that simple. Focus on the list and balancing the scale of how many Eats you eat in a day versus Cheats. You can do this and you are going to do this. You don't need to worry about fat, fibre, calories or anything other than what you've learned. And, most importantly, remember that when you focus on eating the Eats, the Cheats take care of themselves. You can do this. **And you will! This is the year.**

Appendix

Cheat Lifestyle Programme for Athletes

If you're an athlete working out more than the average person, The Cheats and Eats Lifestyle Programme changes in terms of diet. How you alter the plan is ultimately dependent on your goals, but if you want to lose weight the plan won't change all that much. (However, if you're interested in improving performance goals, you might need to change the plan further.)

First, if you are an athlete you may need to eat more. If you find that you don't have the energy to do your normal workout routine or regular activities, try increasing the amount of non-starchy vegetables that you eat. These are Eats so it really doesn't have that big of effect on the diet or number of Cheats you use each day. If that doesn't work, increase the amount of starchy carbohydrates you eat.

Because athletes work out harder and longer than most people, their workouts tend to deplete more sugar reserves. Eating about another 100g extra of starchy carbohydrates, like beans, during a meal will provide the replenishment those glycogen stores need. Seeds and nuts are your friend here. Use these nutrient boosters as well.

It can also be helpful to eat more protein at certain times of the day. If you eat breakfast at 8 a.m., have lunch at noon, and then eat dinner at 6 p.m. or later, drinking a protein shake around 3 or 4 p.m. in the afternoon can help ensure that your body is getting enough protein to recover and maintain the improvements in performance that your workouts should create.

However, the afternoon "snack shake" shouldn't become a meal, because that adds too many calories to your daily diet and will counteract any benefit you get from the protein. The snack shake should simply be made of protein; no fat and no carbs are necessary. Consuming just protein at this time in the day will stimulate your fat-burning mode whereas having a full meal in shake form will only tell the body that it should store any excess calories as fat (exactly the opposite of what you want for effective weight loss!).

This is only relevant to athletes. An increase in protein for the average person, uncoupled with exercise, will not help you lose weight or build muscle. At best, it will be a neutral meal. At worst, the protein will be so unnecessary that all of it will just be oxidised for energy, offsetting the energy that might have been burned from fat. The point is that you only need to eat extra protein throughout the day if you create a deficit – in other words, if you have a well-established base fitness and do hard, long or intense workouts.

Three Other Foods That Could be Holding You Back

In addition to the foods restricted on the Cheats list, there are three other foods that sometimes restrict weight loss: beans and pseudo-seeds like quinoa, smoked foods and healthy fats.

Beans and Pseudo-Seeds like Quinoa

If you're having trouble losing weight, it could be the beans or the seeds. Though technically these foods are free, many people don't digest these foods well so very large portions can hold you back from losing weight. Try eliminating beans from your diet and see if it helps. If it does, consider beans and seeds as Cheats.

Smoked Foods

Smoked foods – from barbecue to smoked salmon – can be high in compounds called polycyclic aromatic hydrocarbons or PAIIs. These compounds are toxic and cause a number of health problems. In general, smoked fish is less healthy for you than unsmoked fish – so if you're struggling with your weight, try eliminating all smoked foods from your diet.

Healthy Fats

If you're struggling with your weight, it can be helpful to avoid eating too many high-fat foods such as nuts, seeds and coconut milk. Though all of these foods contain healthy fats that are good for you, it's still fat – which your body may be storing instead of burning – especially if you're not following the Exercise Plans from Chapter 3.

However, it's important to still include a healthy fat in each meal – so that you will feel satiated and be able to wait for your next meal to eat again.

Useful Measurements

FOR 100 CALORIES CHEATS
(the household measures are an average, estimated guidance).

Food	Household measure	Grams
Bread	1 large slice	40g
Bagel	Half bagel	40g
Dark rye bread	¾ slice	50g
Pasta (cooked)	6 tbsp	100g
Pasta (raw)	2 tbsp	30g
Rice (cooked)	6 tbsp	80g
Rice (raw)	2 tbsp	30g
Crackers	3	21g
Oven chips (thick cut)	8	65g
French fries	Small handful	45g
Pizza	1 slice	50g
Granola	Small handful	25g
Popcorn		20g
Fruit snack bars		25g
Teacake	Half	30g
Scone	Half	30g
Croissant	Half	30g
Cream cake	Half	30g
Chocolate (dark 70% cocoa)	2 large squares	20g
Chocolate (milk)		20g
Milk (whole)		150ml

Food	Household measure	Grams
Milk (semi-skimmed)		200ml
Milk (skimmed)		250ml
Cheddar cheese	Match box size	25g
Feta/halloumi	Match box size	30g
Butter	1 tbsp	15g
Cream (single)	2½ tbsp	45ml
Cream (double)	1 tbsp	15ml
Crème fraiche	2 tbsp	30ml
Crème fraiche (reduced fat)	4 tbsp	60ml
Ice cream (non-dairy)	2 scoop	90ml
Ice cream (dairy)	1 scoop	45ml
Soya milk		250ml
Nut milk		300ml
Cream cheese (full fat)	¼ (180g) pack	45g
Cream cheese (half fat)	¼ (180g) pack	45g
Yogurt (0% fat)	6 tbsp	200g
Yogurt (low fat)	4 tbsp	150g
Yogurt (full fat)	3 tbsp	100g
Sweetcorn (tinned)	5 tbsp	130g
Oats (raw)	2 tbsp	30g
Pearl barley (raw)	2 tbsp	30g
Pearl barley (cooked)	6 tbsp	100g
Bulgur wheat (raw)	2 tbsp	30g
Bulgur wheat (cooked)	6 tbsp	100g
Spelt (raw)	2 tbsp	30g
Spelt (cooked)	6 tbsp	100g
Oysters	8 oysters	120g
Offal (liver)		120g

Food	Household measure	Grams
Veal (lean)		100g
Sausage (pork, reduced fat)	1 sausage	50g
Bacon (back, fat trimmed)	2 rashers	60g
Ham (finely sliced)		60g
Tofu		100g
Edamame	3 tbsp	80g
Nut butters	1 heaped tbsp	20g
Wine	1 small glass	125ml
Beer	1 small glass	250ml
Spirits	1½ shots	50ml
Fruit sauces (condiments, branded)	3 heaped tbsp	60g
Chutney (fruit/onion, branded)	2 heaped tbsp	40g
Bearnaise/hollandaise (branded)	2 heaped tbsp	50g
Gravy (fresh)		200ml
Dips (pulses, branded) e.g. hummus	2 heaped tbsp	40g
Reduced fat dips (pulses, branded) e.g. hummus	2½ heaped tbsp	50g
Dips (yogurt or vegetables) e.g. Tzatziki	3 heaped tbsp	65g
BBQ/Hoisin/plum sauce (branded)	5 tbsp	75g
Jam (branded)	1½ tsp	45g
Jelly (made up, branded)		200g
Ketchup (branded)	6½ tbsp	100g

Food	Household measure	Grams
Mayo (branded)	1 tbsp	15g
Mayo (reduced fat, branded)	2 heaped tbsp	40g
Beef, mince (raw, 10% fat)	⅛ 500g pack	60g
Beef, mince (raw, 5% fat)	⅙ 500g pack	80g
Beef, fillet steak (raw)	Pack of cards size	100g
Beef, rib eye (raw)	½ pack of cards size	50g
Chicken breast (raw)	Palm-sized fillet	100g
Chicken breast (raw, with skin)	Small palm-sized fillet	70g
Chicken thigh (raw, boneless)	2 small thighs	70g
Chicken drumstick (raw, with bone)	2 small drumsticks	70g
Lamb, mince (raw)	⅛ 400g pack	50g
Pork, mince (raw, lean)	⅛ 500g pack	60g
Lamb, shoulder (raw, edible portion)	½ pack of cards size	50g
Pork fillet (raw, lean)	Pack of cards size	100g
Salmon fillet (boneless, skinless, raw)	Small palm-sized fillet	60g
Tuna steak (raw)	Pack of cards size	100g
White fish (boneless, skinless, raw)	Pack of cards size	100g
Anchovy fillets (tinned)	⅓ tin	40g
Mackerel fillet (boneless, skinless, raw)	Pack of cards size	100g
Ravioli (fresh, meat filled)	⅕ 250g pack	50g
Ravioli (fresh, mozzarella)	⅕ 250g pack	50g

Food	Household measure	Grams
Crisps	1 small handful	20g
Breakfast cereal (sweet e.g. cheerios)		25g
Breakfast cereal (high-fibre)		30g
Eggs	1 extra large or 2 small	70g
Nuts	1 small handful	25g

Bibliography

1. Dallman, M. et al. "Chronic stress and obesity: A new view of 'comfort food.'" *PNAS*, (2003) Vol. 100, pp. 11696–11701.
2. Epel ES, McEwen B, Seeman T, et al. "Stress and body shape: Stress-induced cortisol secretion is consistently greater among women with central fat". *Psychosom Med*, (2000) 62(5): 623–632.
3. Jackson SE, Kirschbaum C, Steptoe A. "Hair cortisol and adiposity in a population-based sample of 2,527 men and women aged 54 to 87years". *Obesity*, (2017) Mar, 25(3): 539–544
4. Epel E, Lapidus R, McEwen B, Brownell K. "Stress may add bite to appetite in women: A laboratory study of stress-induced cortisol and eating behaviour". *Psychoneuroendocrinology*, (2001) 26(1): 37–49.
5. Ledikwe J.H., Blanck H.M., Khan L.K., Serduna M.K., Seymour J.D., Tohill B.C., Rolls B.J. "Dietary energy density is associated with energy intake and weight status in US adults". *Am J Clin Nutr*, (2006) Vol 83(6): 1362–1368
6. Yihai Cao. "Angiogenesis modulates adipogenesis and obesity". *J Clin Invest.* (2007) Spe 4;117(9): 2362–2368
7. Fuhrman J., Sarter B., Glaser D., Acocella S. "Changing perceptions of hunger on a high nutrient density diet". *Nutr J* (2010) (9):51
8. Lichtman, S. W., Pisarska, K., Berman, E. R., Pestone, M., Dowling, H., Offenbacher, E. and Heymsfield, S. B. "Discrepancy between self-reported and actual caloric intake and exercise in obese subjects". *New England Journal of Medicine*, (1992) 327(27), 1893–1898

9. Ello-Martin, J. A., Ledikwe, J. H., and Rolls, B. J. "The influence of food portion size and energy density on energy intake: implications for weight management". *The American journal of clinical nutrition*, (2005) 82(1), 236S–241S.

10. Kral, T. V., and Rolls, B. J. "Energy density and portion size: their independent and combined effects on energy intake". *Physiology and behaviour*, (2004) 82(1), 131–138.

11. Wansink, B., Painter, J. E., and North, J. "Bottomless Bowls: Why Visual Cues of Portion Size May Influence Intake**". *Obesity Research*, (2005) 13(1), 93–100.

12. Rodriguez-Hernandez H., Simental-Mendia L.E., Rodriguez-Ramirez G., Reyes-Romero M.A. "Obesity and inflammation: epidemiology, risk factors, and markers of inflammation". *Int J Endocrinol*. 2013; 2013: 678159.

13. Martin, S. S., Qasim, A., and Reilly, M. P. "Leptin Resistance: A Possible Interface of Inflammation and Metabolism in Obesity-Related Cardiovascular Disease". *Journal of the American College of Cardiology*, (2008) 52(15), 1201–1210

14. Vasunilashorn, S. "Retrospective Reports of Weight Change and Inflammation in the US National Health and Nutrition Examination Survey". *Journal of Obesity*, (2013), 601534.

15. Yao, M., and Roberts, S. B. "Dietary energy density and weight regulation". *Nutrition reviews*, (2001) 59(8), 247–258

16. Parretti, H. M., Aveyard, P., Blannin, A., Clifford, S. J., Coleman, S. J., Roalfe, A. and Daley, A. J. "Efficacy of water preloading before main meals as a strategy for weight loss in primary care patients with obesity: RCT". Obesity, (2015) 23: 1785–1791.

17. Kowalczyk M.C., Kowalczyk P., Tolstykh O., et al. "Synergistic effects of combined phytochemicals and skin cancer prevention in SENCAR mice". *Cancer Prev Res*. (2010) 3(2): 170–178.

18. Bell, E. A., and Rolls, B. J. "Energy density of foods affects energy intake across multiple levels of fat content in lean and obese women". *The American journal of clinical nutrition*, (2001) 73(6), 1010–1018.

19. Xu X., Yu E., Gao X., Song N., Liu L., Wei X., Zhang W., Fu C. "Red and processed meat intake and risk of colorectal

adenomas: a meta-analysis of observational studies". *Int J Cancer*. (2013) Jan 15;132(2):437-48

20. Moorhead, S. A., Welch, R. W., Barbara, M., Livingstone, E., McCourt, M., Burns, A. A., and Dunne, A. "The effects of the fibre content and physical structure of carrots on satiety and subsequent intakes when eaten as part of a mixed meal". *British Journal of Nutrition*, (2006) 96(03), 587–595.

21. Wing, R. R., Jeffery, R. W., Burton, L. R., Thorson, C., Sperber Nissinoff, K., and Baxter, J. E. "Food provision vs structured meal plans in the behavioral treatment of obesity". *International journal of obesity*, (1996) 20(1), 56–62.

22. Rolls, B. J., Castellanos, V. H., Halford, J. C., Kilara, A., Panyam, D., Pelkman, C. L., Thorwart, M. L. "Volume of food consumed affects satiety in men". *The American journal of clinical nutrition*, (1998) 67(6), 1170–1177.

23. Hursel R., Viechtbauer W., Westerterp-Plantenga M.S. "The effects of green tea on weight loss and weight maintenance: a meta-analysis". *International Journal of Obesity*, (2009) 33(9): 956–961.

24. Parvez S., Malik K.A., Ah Kang S., Kim H.Y. "Probiotics and their fermented food products are beneficial for health". *J Appl Microbiol*. (2006) 100(6): 1171–1185.

25. Daubenmier J.1., Kristeller J., Hecht F.M., Maninger N., Kuwata M., Jhaveri K., Lustig R.H., Kemeny M., Karan L., Epel E. "Mindfulness Intervention for Stress Eating to Reduce Cortisol and Abdominal Fat among Overweight and Obese Women: An Exploratory Randomized Controlled Study". *J Obes*. (2011); 2011: 651936

Index

ALA fatty acids 44
alcohol 40, 87, 98, 99
allergies 50
amino acids 46, 50
angiogenesis inhibitors 34
antioxidants 30, 40, 102
appetite
    factors affecting 16, 98
    regulation 39
appetizer recipes 261–267
athletes
    Cheat and Eats Lifestyle
    Program for 290–291
    flow state 58

B vitamins 30
bacon 48
beans 88, 291
    soaking and cooking 149
bedtime, eating before 98
beef 48
belly fat 14, 16, 61, 108
    cortisol and 16, 61
black tea 86, 102
blender 137
blood sugar 16, 35, 45, 46,
    47, 61, 110
brain 20, 280
    brain chaos 19, 20
    brain chemicals 56
    effect of sugar on 45
    hunger signals 4, 16, 23,
    29–30, 46
    mindful eating 107–108
    rewiring 8, 25, 43, 151
    stress and 61, 63
bread 8
breakfast 99
    cultural differences 150,
    151
    meal replacement shakes
    99
    power breakfasts
    166–167
    recipes 153–167
    skipping 99
    smoothies 47

switching size and foods
    100

caffeine 40, 102
calories 28, 32, 110
can't-get-full feeling 14
carbohydrates 15, 30, 45, 46
cardiovascular workouts
    65–66
catechins 102
change
    gradual 8, 13, 20, 24–25
    "one thing" exercise
    24–25, 287–288
Cheat Confetti 149–150,
    190–191
Cheat Cuts 101, 102, 120
cheatifying recipes 146
Cheats
    100 Calorie Cheats 84,
    293–297
    "banking" 103, 105–106,
    282
    on the Cheat Sheet 87,
    89, 91, 93
    daily allowance 84, 111
    earning extra 95, 118,
    119–120, 125, 128, 133
    Eats become Cheats 95,
    103
    limiting 36–38, 42, 84,
    103–104
    regular consumption 83
Cheats and Eats Exercise
    Plan 53–79
    building your base 54–56,
    282–283
    charting progress 55,
    112–113
    finding the exercise you
    love 54, 57–61, 283
    fitness fusion 53–65
    flow 57–61, 67
    four pillars of 54–65
    fun activities 56
    little and often 55
    social cardio 67

stress, confronting 61–64
Three-Week Plan 66–79,
    118, 126, 133
time management 55
Cheats and Eats Lifestyle
Program
    for athletes 290–291
    change, gradual 8, 13, 22,
    24–25
    diet fusion 41
    doable 5, 13, 41, 52, 82,
    286–287
    feedback 7, 13, 18, 21, 22,
    24, 82, 83, 94, 106, 109
    flexibility 8, 29
    frequently asked
    questions 101–105
    long-term health benefits
    104
    maintenance plan
    278–289
    making it work for you
    23–24
    math of 94
    for men 105
    setbacks 106, 128, 287
    simplicity of 5, 6, 22, 41,
    51, 84, 287
    suitability for everyone
    6–7
    three pillars of 29–40
    Three-Week Lifestyle
    Program Plan 110–133
    transition period 127
    typical plate of food
    43–44, 51, 94, 111
Cheats and Eats Sheet 5, 22,
    83, 84, 86–94
chia seeds 43, 119, 120
chicken 48–49
cholesterol 44
    VLDL cholesterol 46
cleaning out cupboards and
    fridge 136
coconut milk 291
coconut oil 44, 147
coffee 86, 95, 102

condiments and sauces 92, 93, 139–140, 253–254
containers, freezer-safe 137
cooking 100–101, 112, 144–150
  basics 146–150
  Magic Fridge 134–141
  Magic Kitchen 145–146
  no-cook meals 102, 111
  recipes see recipes
corn 28, 48, 91, 103
corn syrup 103
cortisol 14–17, 38, 43, 61, 65, 110
  belly fat and 15, 16, 61
  exercise and 60, 61
  reduction 29, 108, 601
  stress and 15, 16, 61
cravings 108–109, 136
CrossFit exercise programmes 12
cutting boards and knives 137

daily activities, exercise as 57
dairy products 31, 87
dancing 58, 126
dessert recipes 268–275
DHA fatty acids 44, 105, 112
diets
  fad diets 2, 12
  failed 2, 11, 12
  magic-bullet solutions 12, 20
  restriction and regimentation 6, 13, 27, 28, 41
  spectrum of 5, 27–28
  see also Cheats and Eats Lifestyle Program
digestion 32
dinner 151
  recipes 204–261
doctor, consulting before exercise 66
drinks
  on the Cheat Sheet 86, 87
  recipes 276–277

eating out 34, 106–107, 146
  "pick your pleasure" 107
Eats
  on the Cheat Sheet 86, 88, 90, 92
  first-serving Eats 95, 103

unlimited 33, 36, 50–51, 83, 84, 95–96, 110, 282
eggs 49
  egg-based breakfasts 162–165
  hard-boiled 147–148
elimination diets 28, 41
emails to yourself 133
energy
  density 31, 32, 33
  eating for energy 110–111
  sources 15, 30
EPA fatty acids 44, 105, 112
exercise
  cortisol and 15, 60, 61
  finding what you love 54, 57–61, 283
  pain 66
  see also Cheats and Eats Exercise Plan; workouts

fad diets 2, 12
fat, body 34, 39, 40, 46
  belly fat 14, 16, 61, 108
  fat cells 39
  storage 16, 29, 39, 61
fat-burning 33–34, 60, 61, 290
fats, dietary 15, 30
  on the Cheat Sheet 90, 91
  healthy fats 40, 43–44, 48, 90, 95, 96, 292
fibre 32, 45, 46, 95
fight or flight response 15
fish 49
  oily 44, 50, 105, 112
  smoked 292
  toxins in 49
fish oil 43
fitness
  30-second chair test 54–55
  building your base 54–56, 282–283
  fitness fusion 53–65
  see also Cheats and Eats Exercise Plan
fitness trackers 112
flaxseeds 43, 120
flow of body and mind 57–61, 67
  stages of 59–60
food chain 49
food diaries 113
food sensitivities 50

French fries 43
fridge
  cleaning out 136
  must-have foods 138–140
  see also Magic Fridge
frozen meals 102
frozen vegetables 102, 139
fruits 95
  on the Cheat Sheet 88
  limiting 103
fullness, feeling of 33, 44, 46, 83, 96, 97, 104

G BOMBS 33, 146
ghrelin 47
ginger 128
glucose 15, 16, 30, 45, 46, 61
gluten-free products 87
glycogen 45
goals 59
  unrealistic 14
good decisions 43, 96
grains, on the Cheat Sheet 90, 91
green tea 102
greens 119–120, 137, 139
  cooking 148
  pre-washed 101
gut bacteria 105

habits, changing 8, 17, 24–25
heart disease 44, 46
heart rate 67, 113
high fructose corn syrup 103
high-nutrient eating 29–36, 41, 96, 97, 104
homeostasis 12, 13, 39
hormones 15, 23, 27, 37, 38, 39, 46, 47
  exercise and 61
  stress hormones 15, 64
  see also cortisol; ghrelin; insulin; leptin
hunger
  assessing 108
  pangs 4, 16, 23, 29–30, 46
  toxic hunger 35

"if only" statements 20
immune system 39
imperfection, acceptance of 24
inflammation 16, 28, 29, 39–40, 41, 45, 50
  acute/chronic 39

anti-inflammatory diets 40
reducing 44, 105
and weight gain 39
injury
avoidance of 58, 67
inflammation and 39
insulin 15, 16, 35, 45, 46, 47
iron 30
isoflavones 50

joints, mobilising 56, 67
junk food 103
"just this once" mentality 13–14, 42

kale 97
kitchen tools 136–138

leptin 39
liver (organ) 45, 46
low glycaemic load 40
lunch 151
recipes 167–204

macronutrients 30, 44
Magic Fridge 134–141
Magic Kitchen 145–146
magnesium 30
maintenance of weight loss 278–289
mantras 125, 288
meal replacement shakes 99
see also shakes and smoothies
meals
go-to meals 112
meal plans 113–117, 121–125, 129–132
no-cook meals 102, 111
standbys 135
switching 100, 151
three meals a day 98–100
meat 48–49
processed meat 48
red meat 48
Mediterranean diet 40
men, Cheat System for 105
metabolism 39, 66
metabolic dysfunction 35
micronutrients 29, 30–31, 32, 33, 36, 110, 282
mindful eating 107–108
Monday morning derailment 6, 13–14
monounsaturated fats 43–44
motivation 3, 12, 18, 27

muscles 43, 65–66
complementary muscles 283
flexibility and strength 56
lean muscle mass 61, 66
mushrooms 34
must, power of 17, 18

negativity 279–280
night-time eating 36, 98
nutrient deficiency 28
nuts and nut butters 92, 93

obesity dilemma, global 45
"obligation meals" 5, 23, 37
obsession with weight loss 18, 19
oils, cooking 146–147
olive oil 44, 147
omega 3 fatty acids 40, 43, 48, 49, 105, 112, 119
omega 6 fatty acids 40, 44, 49
organic food 49, 90, 102, 139
oven baked and casseroles, recipes 228–242

Paleo diet 12, 13
pea and rice protein 50
peanuts 103
PEERtrainer 4, 5
phytonutrients 30, 40, 51
pilates 65, 67
pizza 12, 30, 108, 134–135
polycyclic aromatic hydrocarbons (PAHs) 291
portion control 3, 27, 28, 41, 96
failure of 29–30, 37–38, 41
portion distortion 37
positivity 280–281
power breakfasts 166–167
pregnancy, weight loss after 4, 37
probiotics 105
processed foods 32, 45, 48, 103
protein 15, 44, 46–50, 95, 96, 291
animal sources 46, 47, 48–49
on the Cheat Sheet 90, 91
plant sources 46–47
protein powders 47, 50, 94

protein shakes 291
pseudo-seeds 291

quinoa 46, 148–149

raw foods 27, 28
recipes
appetizers 261–267
breakfasts 153–167
Cheat Confetti 190–191
cheatifying 146
desserts 268–275
dinners 204–261
drinks 276–277
high nutrient eats 255–261
lunches 167–204
oven baked and casseroles 228–242
protein based 192–204, 243–253
salads and dressings 173–190
sauces 253–254
slow cooker and stews 224–228
soups 167–171, 172, 204–215, 217–223, 225–226
relaxation exercises 63, 65
restaurant meals see eating out
restrictive diets 6, 13, 27, 28, 41
rice cooker 137
roap map 23
running 58, 61

salad bowls 34, 35, 137–138
salads and dressings, recipes 173–190
salmon 49, 151
salt 45, 103
satiation point 45
satiety see fullness, feeling of
setbacks 2, 3, 13, 23, 42, 106, 128, 287
shakes and smoothies 47, 139, 153–161, 290
skin ageing 46
sleep 65
amount of 65
healthy sleep patterns 65
slow cooker and stews, recipes 224–228
smoked foods 103, 291
smoothies see shakes and

smoothies
snacking 46, 87, 98, 99
  late-night 98
soft drinks 87
soup recipes 167–171, 172,
  204–215, 217–223,
  225–226
soy protein 50
soy and soy-based products
  90, 103
spices 92, 93, 128–129,
  139–140
  shortcuts 140–141
sports 61, 118, 283
starving yourself 5, 12, 34
stress 3, 14, 15, 61–64
  chronic 15, 16
  confronting 61–64
  cortisol and 15, 16, 61
  health, impact on 15
  management 16, 62, 63
  mental 61
  physiological 61
substitution foods 108–109,
  134
sucrose 46
sugar 30, 32, 45–46, 89,
  103, 109
  cutting down on 45, 46
  substitutes 109
  sugar rush 46
  see also sweeteners
sugar, blood see blood sugar
supplements 44, 49, 50,
  104–105, 112
sweeteners
  artificial 89, 101–102,
  109
  natural 45, 89
swimming 133

taste buds, changing 102,
  127
Three-Week Lifestyle
  Program Plan 110–133
  exercise plans 118, 126,
  133
  meal plans 113–117,
  121–125, 129–132
  Week One 110–118
  Week Two 119–126
  Week Three 127–133
Three-Week Workout Plan
  66–79
  warming up/cooling
  down 67–68
  Week One 68–71, 118

Week Two 72–73, 126
  Week Three 74–78, 133
toxic hunger 35
trigger foods 136, 150
triglycerides 30, 45
turmeric 128

veganism 12, 41, 47, 105
vegetable-only diets 27, 28
vegetables
  on the Cheat Sheet 86
  filling power 33, 35,
  96–97, 104
  frozen 102, 139
  greens 119–120, 137, 139
  nutrient-dense 29, 31, 32,
  40, 96–97
  unlimited 86, 95–96

walking 54, 55, 56–57, 59,
  60, 67, 112, 118
water intake 43
weighing yourself 118, 284
weight gain
  cortisol and 15, 16
  inflammation and 39
weight loss
  after pregnancy 4, 37
  maintaining 278–289
  psychology of 21
  struggles with 12, 14, 15,
  21, 26–27, 53
  temporary 28
  three essential pillars of
  29–40
weight, perfect 283
wheat products 87
whey protein 50
willpower 23, 27, 96, 111,
  136
wine 29, 87, 99
workouts 6, 12, 14, 43,
  53, 54
  cardiovascular 65–66
  flow states 58, 60
  resistance based 66
  skipping 64, 282
  weight-lifting 65, 66
  see also Three-Week
  Workout Plan

yeast products 87
yoga 61, 65, 67, 282

zumba 61, 67